"We are already hugely indebted to Christfried Toegel for his numerous and crucial contributions to Freud scholarship, above all the first complete edition of anything Freud published during his lifetime. Here, Toegel is setting the record straight: Despite frequent claims to Freud's 'hidden' or 'repressed' religiosity, he minutely traces the development of Freud's unabashed, unwavering, and indeed un-ambivalent 'absolutely negative attitude towards all religion.' Indispensable reading for anyone seeking an accurate understanding of Freud and, in a broader context, the uneasy relationship between science and religion."

Ernst Falzeder, former senior research fellow at University College London (retired), editor of Freud/Abraham and Freud/Ferenczi correspondence, author of *Psychoanalytic Filiations: Mapping the Psychoanalytic Movement*

"*Freud Against God* takes us on a chronological guided tour through the landscape of Freud's disbelief, beginning with the two-year-old infant preaching on 'God Almighty' and ending with the 82-year-old Professor stating his 'absolutely negative attitude toward any religion'. There has never been any doubt about Freud's antipathy towards religion, but it has often been obscured by other details of his life and work, or even overlooked. By bringing together a lifetime's scattered comments Christfried Toegel underlines the fundamental importance of that 'negative attitude' in Freud's science and life. There could be no better guide to this territory than Christfried Toegel. Over the past four decades his books and articles have greatly expanded the range of Freud biography. This concise study offers the newcomer an excellent overview of the theme: scholars familiar with the biographies will find here a useful compendium of references to the lifelong duel between Freud and religion."

Michael Molnar, an archivist, researcher and Director of the Freud Museum London between 1986 and 2009, he edited Freud's 1929–1939 diary notes and wrote *Looking through Freud's Photos*, a study of Freud's photo library, and has published numerous articles on Freud biography

"In famously characterising himself as 'a completely godless Jew' to his friend the Swiss pastor Oskar Pfister, Freud was not joking. He was a thoroughgoing atheist, who rarely lost an opportunity to challenge the illusions of religion, though he could see – and was not without compassion towards – how comforting these might be. In this succinct and eminently readable volume, leading international Freud scholar Chris Toegel guides the reader through Freud's life and writings revealing in great clarity the key successive encounters he had with religion and religious belief. Toegel lets Freud speak, quoting his actual words extensively, thus leaving us in no doubt what the Professor actually thought and his still radical and trenchant proposals for policy and social reform in this area. With the place of religion in modern civil society remaining a highly contested subject, this unsparing volume will be an invaluable read for anyone who wants a reliable primer on the foundations of psychoanalytic thinking on god. Challenging, controversial, and eminently readable, *Freud Against God* will no-doubt prove one of the most compelling volumes on the subject. Buy it! Read it!"

Roger Willoughby, Oxford Brookes University, UK, clinical psychologist and historian of psychoanalysis, author of *Masud Khan: The Myth and the Reality* (2005) and *Freud's British Family: Reclaiming Lost Lives in Manchester and London* (2024)

Freud Against God

Freud Against God traces the development of Freud's atheism, from his youth through to *Moses and Monotheism*, published in 1939.

Christfried Toegel takes a largely chronological approach, tracing how biographical developments in Freud's life and political events gradually led to his conviction that it is "a greater risk if we maintain our present attitude to religion than if we give it up." The book considers Freud's life, his writing, and the influence of politics and society. Chapter 1 covers the genesis of Freud's critical attitude towards religion and the influence of Ludwig Börne, Charles Darwin, and John Stuart Mill. Chapter 2 focuses on Freud's critiques of religion in his writing between 1907 and 1939. Chapter 3 describes how Freud dealt with the deaths of his daughter and his grandson, and with cancer and death. Chapter 4 focuses on religion, politics, and society, particularly the role of the Catholic Church in relation to Freud and psychoanalysis.

Written by a leading Freud scholar, this book provides a compact overview of Freud's atheism. *Freud Against God* will be of great interest to academics and scholars of Freud and religion.

Christfried Toegel is one of the leading Freud biographers of our time. He is the editor of the 23-volume Sigmund Freud Complete Edition, the first complete edition of Freud's writings. Among Toegel's more than 150 publications on the history of psychoanalysis and Freud biographies are ten books that have been translated into eight languages.

History of Psychoanalysis
Series Editor
Peter L. Rudnytsky

This series seeks to present outstanding new books that illuminate any aspect of the history of psychoanalysis from its earliest days to the present, and to reintroduce classic texts to contemporary readers.

Other titles in the series:

The Marquis de Puysegur and Artificial Somnambulism
Memoirs to Contribute to the History and Establishment of Animal Magnetism
Edited and translated by Adam Crabtree and Sarah Osei-Bonsu

The Subversive Edge of Psychoanalysis
David James Fisher

The Vicissitudes of Psychoanalysis in Soviet Russia, 1930–1980
Lizaveta van Munsteren

Freud's British Family
Reclaiming Lost Lives in Manchester and London
Roger Willoughby

Sigmund Freud's Inner Divisions
Personal and Theoretical
Ken Fuchsman

Sigmund Freud on the Way to Paris, 1873–1885
Foundations of Psychoanalysis
Giosuè Ghisalberti

Freud Against God
The Development of Sigmund Freud's Atheism
Christfried Toegel

For further information about this series please visit https://www.routledge.com/The-History-of-Psychoanalysis-Series/book-series/KARNHIPSY

Freud Against God

The Development of Sigmund Freud's Atheism

Christfried Toegel

Routledge
Taylor & Francis Group
LONDON AND NEW YORK

First published 2026
by Routledge
4 Park Square, Milton Park, Abingdon, Oxon OX14 4RN

and by Routledge
605 Third Avenue, New York, NY 10158

Routledge is an imprint of the Taylor & Francis Group, an informa business

British Library Cataloguing-in-Publication Data
A catalogue record for this book is available from the British Library

ISBN: 978-1-041-14355-0 (hbk)
ISBN: 978-1-041-14357-4 (pbk)
ISBN: 978-1-003-67404-7 (ebk)

DOI: 10.4324/9781003674047

Typeset in Times New Roman
by Apex CoVantage, LLC

Dedicated to my deceased friend Manfred Wuketits

"... The voice of the intellect is a soft one, but it does not rest till it has gained a hearing"

Sigmund Freud (1927)

Contents

Preface

On the occasion of Sigmund Freud's 150th birthday in 2006, the Catholic Academy of Bavaria invited me to give a lecture on "The Significance of Religion in Sigmund Freud's Life." It was both a success and a disaster. Immediately after receiving the invitation, I took the precaution of calling the then director of studies, Dr. Armin Riedel, to tell him what the audience could expect from the topic. It was not an everyday occurrence for me to speak to an audience at a Catholic academy about the atheism of the Jew Freud. Dr. Riedel was able to convince me that I should not take any false considerations into account. I took this statement at face value, with the result that during my lecture, for the first time in my life, I felt that I could use bodyguards.

This experience made me realize that many people are not completely unemotional about this issue. Therefore, I decided to expand my lecture into a small book. A book has the advantage that the author is usually not directly confronted with a large number of angry readers, but can relatively easily avoid any uproar.

Christfried Toegel
Lausanne, June 2025

Prologue: ". . . exclude all believers . . . from attending university"

> Consistently, one would have to exclude all other believers from attending university [. . .]
>
> *Sigmund Freud*
> *Letter to Theodor Reik from 21 October 1937 (Reik, 1956)*

This book traces the development of Freud's atheism, beginning with his ironic remarks in his youth and ending with his late work *Moses and Monotheism* from 1939.

There is not much in it that others have not said and written before me. Peter Gay in particular has convincingly shown in his book *A Godless Jew* (Gay, 1987) that all attempts to appropriate Freud for one religion or another are unfounded. Nor is it true that Freud's attitude to religion was ambivalent, as is repeatedly claimed (see for example Heine, 2006).

However, my approach differs from Peter Gay's in that I take a largely chronological approach. This makes it particularly clear how biographical developments in Freud's life and political events gradually led to his conviction, that it is "a greater risk if we maintain our present attitude to religion than if we give it up" (Freud, 1927, p. 35).

As he grew older, Freud became tougher and demanded consequences. Two years before his death, at the age of 81, he wrote to Theodor Reik: "To act consistently, one would have to exclude all other believers from attending university [. . .]"(Reik, 1956, S. 655).

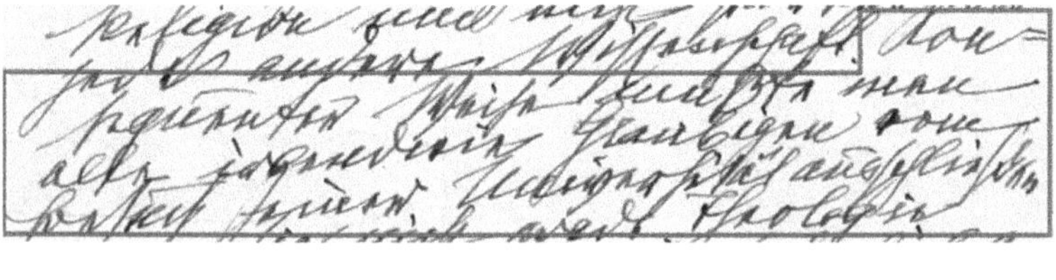

Figure 0.1 Excerpt from Freud's letter to Reik

How can Freud's rejection of all religion be reconciled with the fact, often emphasized by Freud himself, that he always felt himself to be a Jew? Freud himself answered this question several times. In a letter to the members of the Jewish Humanity Association B'nai B'rith, who had congratulated him on his 70th birthday, he wrote on 6 May 1926:

> What tied me to Jewry was – I have to admit it – not the faith, not even the national pride, for I was always an unbeliever, have been brought up without religion, but not without respect for the so-called "ethical" demands of human civilization.
>
> (Freud, 1961, p. 366)

And in response to a letter of welcome sent to Freud by a Zionist organization in 1938 on the occasion of his arrival in the London emigration, we read that he did not want to be treated as a "leader in Israel" and that he had an "absolutely negative attitude towards all religion [. . .]" (Freud, 1954, p. 10).

But as a kind of consolation, as it were, for readers who do not share Freud's view, I would like to add a few remarks about the friendship between Sigmund Freud and the Swiss Protestant pastor Oskar Pfister (1873–1956). At the very beginning of their 30-year correspondence, Freud had written: "I am very much struck by the fact that it never occurred to me how extraordinarily helpful the psycho-analytic method might be in pastoral work, but that is surely accounted for by the remoteness from me, as a wicked pagan, of the whole system of ideas" (Freud and Pfister, 1963, p. 17). Freud's friendly relationship with Pfister had even led him to postpone the publication of his major critical work on religion, *The Future of an Illusion*. In an October 1927 letter, he wrote to Pfister:

> In the next few weeks a pamphlet of mine will be appearing which has a great deal to do with you. I had been wanting to write it for a long time, and postponed it out of regard for you, but the impulse became too strong. The subject-matter – as you will easily guess – is my completely negative attitude to religion, in any form and however attenuated, and, though there can be nothing new to you in this, I feared, and still fear, that such a public profession of my attitude will be painful to you. When you have read it you must let me know what measure of toleration and understanding you are able to preserve for the hopeless pagan.
>
> (Freud and Pfister, 1963, p. 109)

Pfister's response is characteristic of the relationship between the two men:

> As for your anti-religious pamphlet, there is nothing new to me in your rejection of religion. I look forward to it with pleasurable anticipation. A powerful-minded opponent of religion is certainly of more service to it than a thousand useless supporters.
>
> (Freud and Pfister, 1963, p. 110)

1 The genesis of Freud's critical attitude toward religion

1.1 Origin and childhood

1.1.1 "... told us *all about God Almighty*"

Sigmund Freud was born on 6 May 1856 in the small Moravian town of Freiberg, today Příbor in the Czech Republic. His parents came from Galicia – his mother Amalia from Brody and his father Jacob from Tysmenitz, both now in the Ukraine. Sigmund was born an uncle because his father had two grown sons from his first marriage, one of whom was already a father.

Freud's father Jacob, a wool merchant, had grown up in the environment of Eastern European Hasidism, but had not joined any particularly Orthodox movement. His mother Amalia had spent part of her youth in Odessa, which had a duty-free port and was considered cosmopolitan. Both parents identified as Jewish, but they were not considered particularly pious in the family.

It is not surprising, then, what Sigmund's mother later told him about his nanny: She was "an elderly person [. . .], she was always carrying you off to some church; when you returned home you preached and told us all about God Almighty" (Freud, 1985, p. 271). His Jewish parents did not see this as a problem, and so Sigmund's early childhood was not marked by religious conflict.

1.1.2 "Jew! get off the pavement!"

An experience Freud recounted in his book *The Interpretation of Dreams* had a very different effect. During a walk together, his father began a conversation with the following words:

> When I was a young man, he said, "I went for a walk one Saturday in the streets of your birthplace; I was well dressed, and had a new fur cap on my head. A Christian came up to me and with a single blow knocked off my

DOI: 10.4324/9781003674047-1

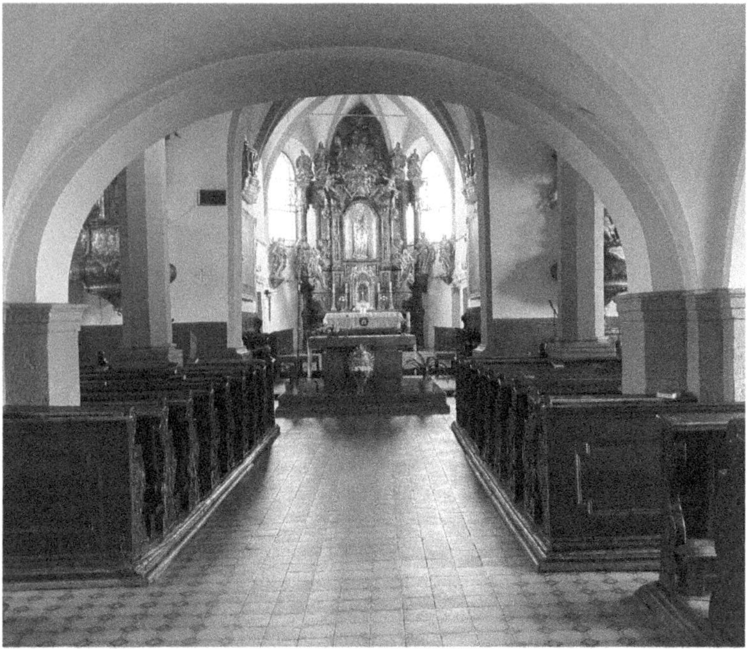

Figure 1.1 Church of the Nativity of the Virgin Mary in Freiberg

> cap into the mud and shouted: "Jew! get off the pavement!" "And what did you do?" I asked. "I went into the roadway and picked up my cap", was his quiet reply. This struck me as unheroic conduct on the part of the big, strong man who was holding the little boy by the hand. I contrasted this situation with another which fitted my feelings better: the scene in which Hannibal's father, Hamilcar Barca, made his boy swear before the household altar to take vengeance on the Romans.
>
> (Freud, 1900, p. 197)

At the time of this conversation with his father Freud was well over ten years old, and he was now developing thoughts of revenge against Christianity, especially the Catholic Church, and identifying himself with Hannibal.

Freud's father, however, was by no means Orthodox. The family tradition has it that he said, "The forest was the first temple of the good Lord!" His grandmother wanted the children to go to synagogue, but he said it was much better if they went to the park and played with him.[1]

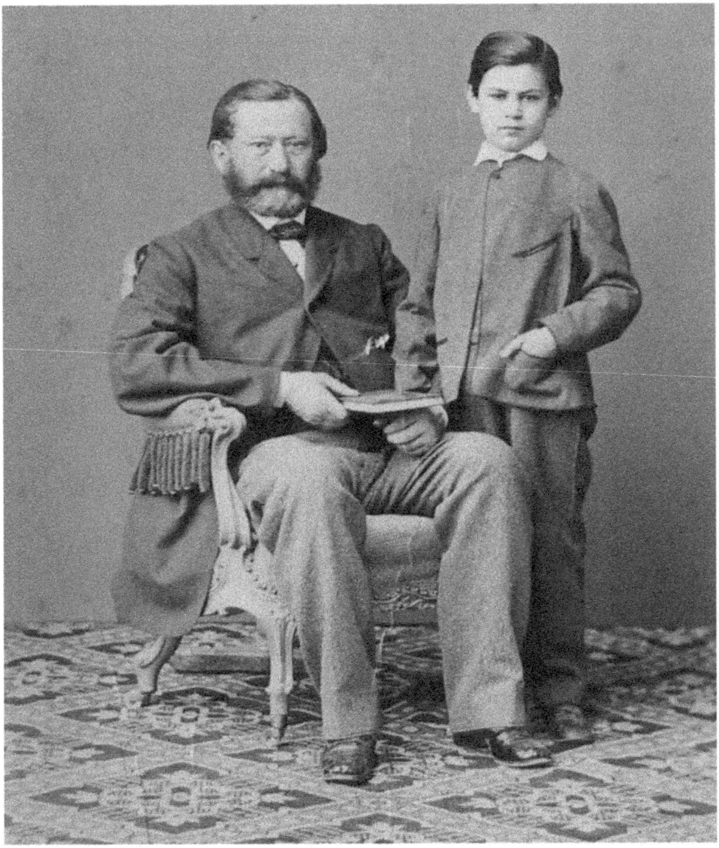

Figure 1.2 Freud and his father, ca. 1865

1.2 Secondary school and university years

1.2.1 Alfred Brehm's illustrated natural history of the animal kingdom

In September 1865, at the age of nine, Freud entered the Realgymnasium. He had presumably not attended school before then, but had received private lessons by his mother.

Natural history, especially vertebrates and invertebrates, was taught in the very first year of the Gymnasium. The teacher was Alois Pokorny (1826–1905). He was the headmaster of the Leopoldstadt Realgymnasium and Freud's most important science teacher. Pokorny was considered a botanist of distinction, and he was a private lecturer at the University of Vienna and co-editor of the *Physiologia plantarum Austriacarum*, published by the Austrian Academy of Sciences in 1873.

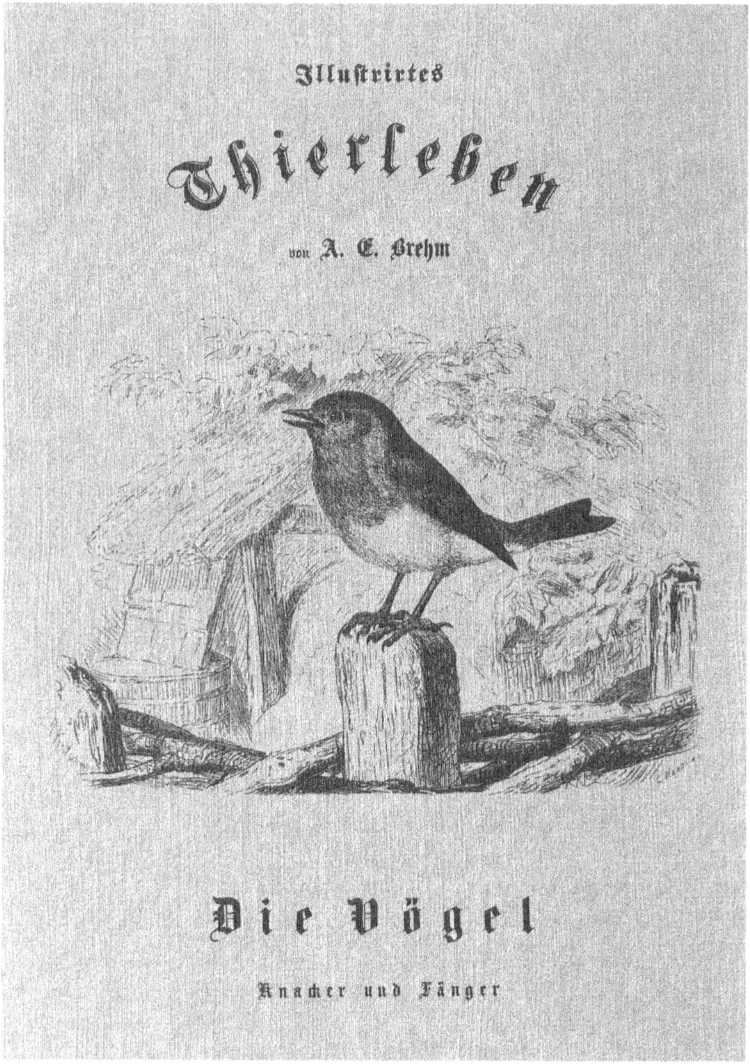

Figure 1.3 Title page of volume 3 of Brehm's "Thierleben"

The students used the sixth edition of Pokorny's *Illustrirter Naturgeschichte des Thierreiches* (*Illustrated Natural History of the Animal Kingdom*) from 1865 as a basis for learning. Freud apparently excelled in this subject, for at the end of the school year he was awarded a prize and presented with a volume of Alfred Brehm's *Geschichte des Tierlebens* (*History of Animal Life*) (Clark, 1980, p. 29; Freud-Bernays, 1989, p. 140). This was presumably the third volume, published in 1866, which, together with the 16 deliveries of the fourth volume still to be published in 1867, was devoted to birds.

In 1867 the focus was on mineralogy and botany, and again a textbook was Pokorny's required reading: *Naturgeschichte des Mineralreiches und Pflanzenreiches* (*Natural History of the Mineral and Plant Kingdoms*). And in 1871, two years before the Matura, zoology was on the curriculum, again taught by Pokorny.

Freud wrote 50 years later about the influence of his teachers:

> It is hard to decide whether what affected us more and was of greater importance to us was our concern with the sciences that we were taught or with the personalities of our teachers. It is true, at least, that this second concern was a perpetual undercurrent in all of us, and that in many of us the path to the sciences led only through our teachers.
>
> (Freud, 1914b, p. 242)

Natural history apparently made such an impression on Freud that he later gave the nickname "Ichthyosaura" – a dinosaur genus from the Cretaceous period – to a girl his friend Eduard was in love with.

1.2.2 Ludwig Börne

On his 13th birthday, 6 May 1869, Freud was given the Viennese edition of the works of Ludwig Börne (1786–1837) in 12 volumes, which he read with "great enthusiasm." The 12 volumes were bound into five books.

The second volume contains a short contribution entitled "O foolish people, O strange world!" The last paragraph of this text reads:

> Religion is love and reconciliation; it is in the word itself: it reunites what was divided. If all men were equally wise, equally gifted, filled with the same inclinations, there would be no need for religion. It is the unity of the manifold, the eternity of the transitory, the gravity of the unjust; it forgives guilt and dissolves sin in the universal light. But what have men made of it! A river of blood flows through eighteen centuries, and Christianity dwells on its banks. How they have profaned the most holy! Religion has been a weapon in the hands of robbers and murderers. How they have degraded the God of Love and misused His teachings as the law of

Figure 1.4 Börne's works in 12 volumes

> their lust for power, as the regulator of their greedy mercenary rights! Has Christianity ever been used for anything other than as an instrument of persecution, if not for the final consolation of defenceless victims? Reconcile its sects, and it faints; destroy Judaism, and it dies. Destroy the religions, and you have destroyed religion. Or is the doctrine of Christ but the tearing ploughshare of mankind? How laborious and painful then was the building up of the land, and until the happy day of the sheaves appears, I cry softly and with a choked voice: O foolish men, O strange world.
>
> (Börne, 1868, vol. 2, p. 125)

Freud had thoroughly read the first two volumes, which were bound together. It should be remembered that Freud received the Börne edition shortly after his father had begun "to take him for walks and to open up to me in conversation his views on the things of this world" (Freud, 1900, p. 197), after the young Sigmund had developed thoughts of revenge against Christianity and identified himself with Hannibal. And it was precisely at this time that he received an edition of Börne, in which Christianity was accused of 1,800 years of bloodshed.

Ludwig Börne was so important to Freud that in the fall of 1885 he was determined to visit Börne's grave in the Père Lachaise cemetery in Paris. But a guide he asked had never heard of Börne, and Freud's "unauthorized search was futile and unsuccessful. At that time, there was no list of the graves of famous people. Today, any visitor can easily find out that Ludwig Börne's grave is in Section 19.

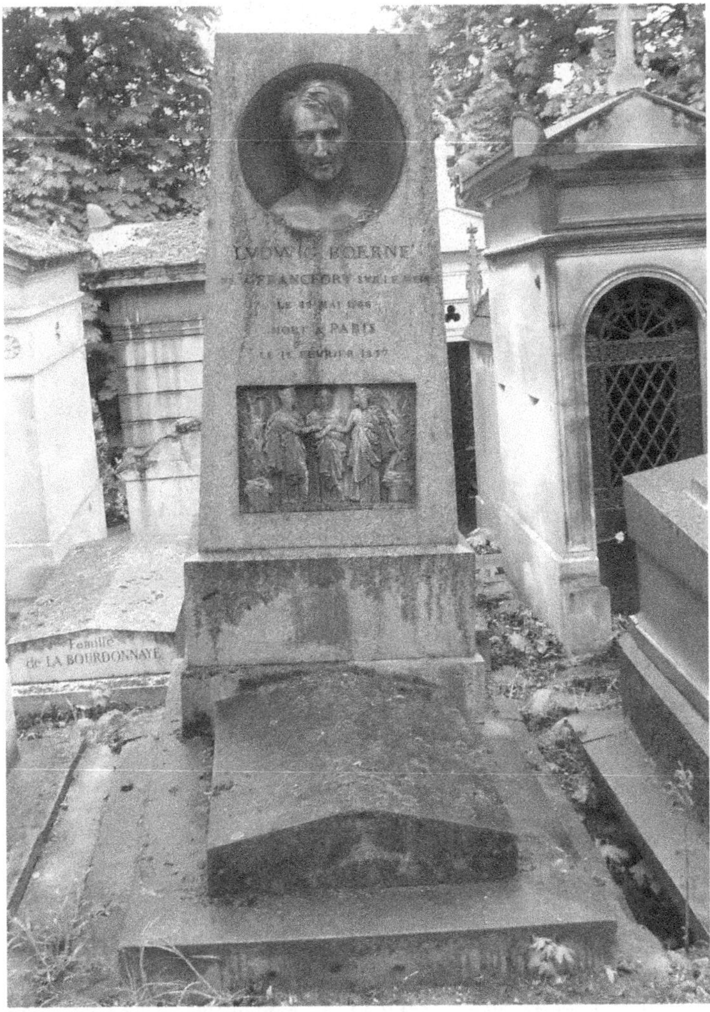

Figure 1.5 Ludwig Börne's grave in Paris

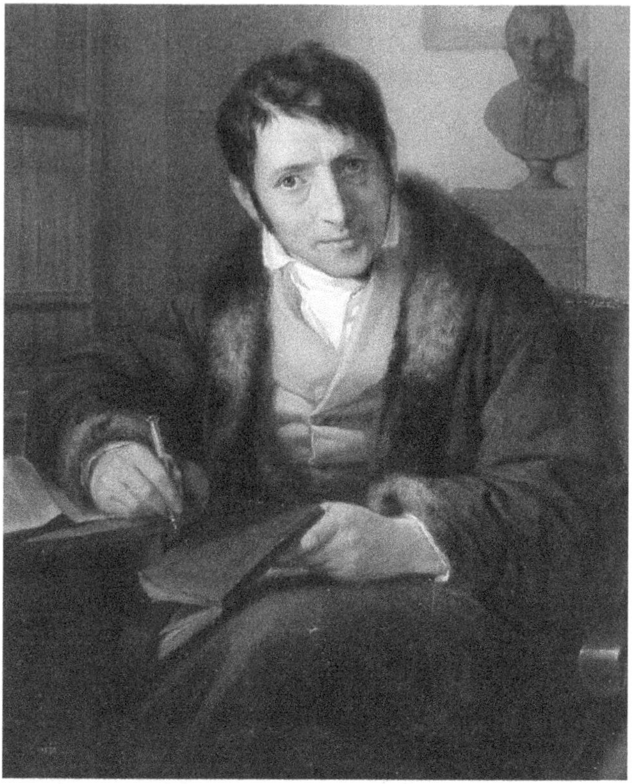

Figure 1.6 Ludwig Börne

And in 1920 Freud wrote that "he had been given Börne's works as a present, that he still possessed the book now, fifty years later, and that it was the only one that had survived from his boyhood" (Freud, 1920, p. 264).

1.2.3 The "Reading Society of German Students in Vienna"

The "Reading Association of German Students in Vienna" (*Leseverein der deutschen Studenten in Wien*) was founded in December 1871. Its aim was "to create a focal point for the entire intellectual life of German students." This was "a real, deep and generally felt need of the German student body."[2] The association was born out of the enthusiasm for the founding of the German Reich, represented a pan-Germanist ideal, and had as its main goal the propagation of the German character of the University of Vienna. The anti-Semitic character of the association's political program was linked to this orientation.

Initially, however, the Reading Society understood anti-Semitism only in a cultural and not in a racial sense (Venturelli, 1984, p. 453). Freud had been a student at the Medical Faculty of the University of Vienna since October 1873 and became a member of the Leseverein during his first year of study, meeting first at Alter Fleischmarkt 16, then at Schönlaterngasse 9, and finally at Wollzeile 33.[3]

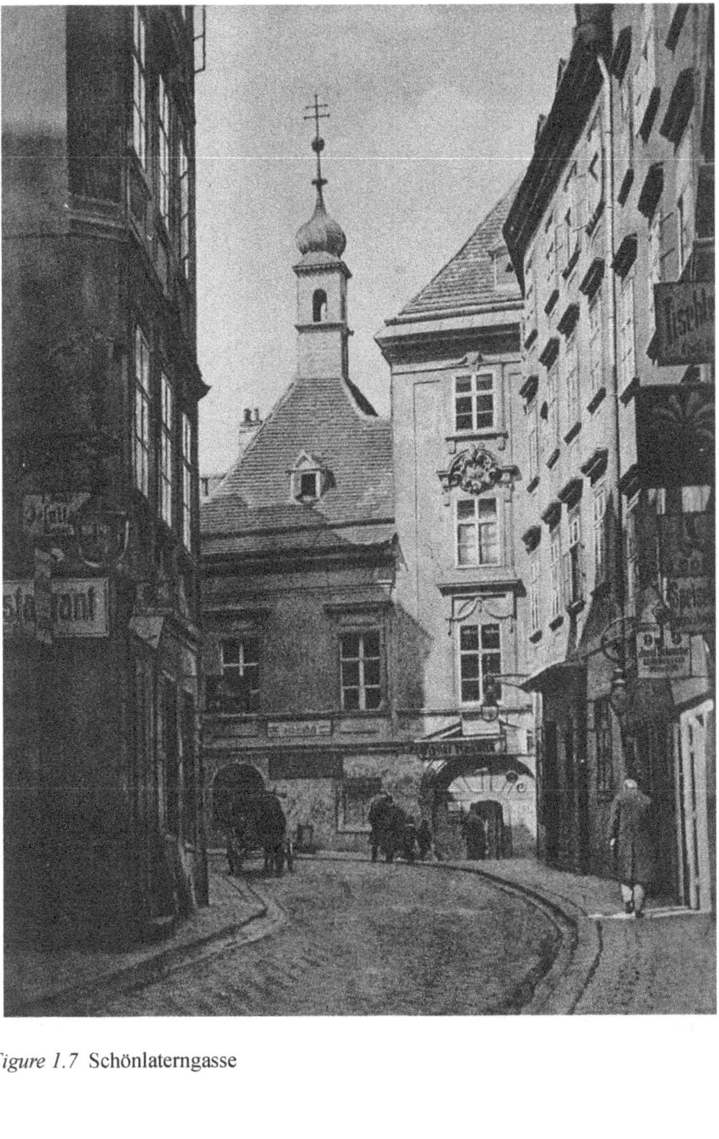

Figure 1.7 Schönlaterngasse

Why does a young, intelligent Jew become a member of an association with an anti-Semitic orientation? One possible answer to this question is the "Jewish self-hatred" thesis (Lessing, 1930).

Freud and other Jewish students of the time were of course well aware of the anti-Jewish tendencies in Vienna. Arthur Schnitzler, who was six years younger than Freud, had also studied medicine in Vienna, as he wrote in his autobiography:

> The German nationalist fraternities had begun to exclude Jews and ethnic Jews from their midst; group clashes during the so-called "Bummel" on Sunday mornings, but also on pub evenings, in the open street between the anti-Semitic fraternities and the free-thinking Landsmannschaften and Corps, some of which consisted largely of Jews [. . .] were not uncommon; challenges between individuals in lecture halls, corridors, and laboratories were the order of the day.
>
> (Schnitzler, 1981, S. 152)

Despite the atmosphere described by Schnitzler, Freud had become a member of the Reading Association of German Students in Vienna. Like him, other young Jewish intellectuals – some only temporarily, however, like Freud's close friend Josef Paneth – who saw their origins as an obstacle to their professional advancement bowed to the pressure to assimilate or even converted to Protestantism or Catholicism. Victor Adler, the son of a Jewish merchant and later the founder of Austrian Social Democracy, was also a member of the Reading Society, was close to the German National Party at the beginning of his political career, and even worked with the anti-Semite Georg von Schönerer on its political program. And Theodor Herzl, the founder of Zionism, was a member of a German nationalist student fraternity.[4] Against this background, Freud's membership in the pan-Germanist anti-Semitic Reading Society was nothing unusual.

Notwithstanding all the attempts to compensate for the apparent or real disadvantages of his own Jewishness through German national activities, Freud probably sensed that the lasting success of such compensation mechanisms and adaptation strategies was very doubtful.

He gradually came to realize that it was more promising to be more efficient than the competition. As a result, Freud began to develop a pronounced ambition and a certain "longing for greatness." In a letter to his fiancée dated 2 February 1886, he formulated his concrete goals as follows:

> I know that [. . .] given favorable conditions I could achieve more than Nothnagel, to whom I consider myself superior, and might possibly reach the level of Charcot.
>
> (Freud, 1961, S. 202)

This is not a particularly modest goal, considering that Hermann Nothnagel was one of the most famous physicians of his time, and Jean-Martin Charcot was considered the leading neuropathologist in Europe; Freud had interned with him at the Paris Salpêtrière for almost six months in 1885/86.

With this idea of greatness, Freud had decided not to allow himself to be assimilated, but to draw attention to himself through achievement. Many years later he explicitly stated that it was the fact that he belonged to Judaism that had a mobilizing effect on his achievement. Looking back, he wrote to Karl Abraham in 1907: "[. . .] that as a Jew you will encounter more difficulties will have the effect, as it has for all of us, of bringing out all of your productive abilities" (Freud and Abraham, 2002, p. 9).

1.2.4 **The Descent of Man** ***and the "airy existence of God"***

Charles Darwin's book *The Descent of Man* was published in London in 1871, and its central claim was that man evolved from higher apes. This was in contrast to the biblical creation story, in which God the Father himself created man from clay. For many believers, Darwin's theory of descent was an affront. An eloquent expression of this horror is the repeatedly circulated exclamation of a bishop's wife: "My dear, let us hope that it is not true, and if it is true, that at least no one will find out!" (Miller, 1924).

Freud had found out. While still at school, he had attended the Sunday lectures of Carl Brühl (1820–1899), who had held the Vienna chair of zoology since 1861 and had become widely known for his popular science lectures. These included "Free Lectures on Darwin's Theory" [. . .] "intended not only to give a definition [. . .] and an account of its significance for natural history, but for the field of knowledge in general, for religion, and for the morals of the human race."[5]

Another of Brühl's lectures dealt with the fragment attributed to Goethe's, the fragment "Nature." He attended this lecture at a time when Freud had to decide what he was going to study. His father had insisted that he follow only his inclinations in choosing a career. Freud wrote about this decision process:

> Neither at that time, nor indeed in my later life, did I feel any particular predilection for the career of a doctor. I was moved, rather, by a sort of curiosity, which was, however, directed more towards human concerns than towards natural objects; [. . .] nor had I grasped the importance of observation as one of the best means of gratifying it. [. . .] At the same time, the theories of Darwin, which were then of topical interest, strongly attracted me, for they held out hopes of an extraordinary advance in our understanding of the world; and it was hearing Goethe's beautiful essay on Nature read aloud at a popular lecture by Professor Carl Brühl just before I left school that decided me to become a medical student.
>
> (Freud, 1925a, p. 8)

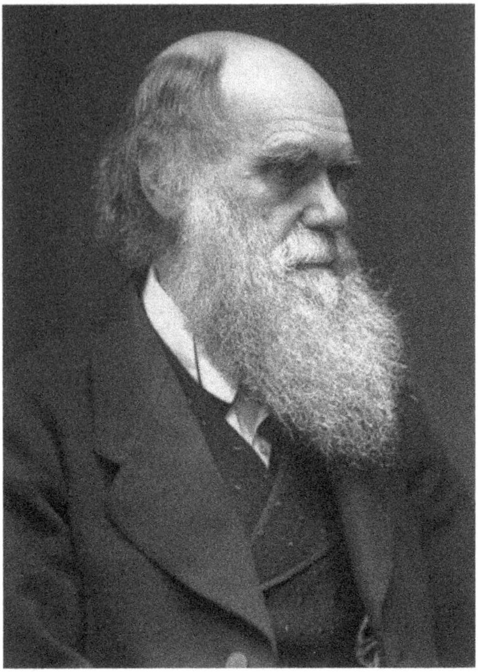

Figure 1.8 Darwin, ca. 1874

At the very beginning of his studies, in the fall of 1873, Freud attended a lecture by Carl Claus on the subject: "General Zoology in Connection With a Critical Presentation of Darwinism." And in 1875 – only five years after the publication of Darwin's *Descent of Man* – Freud bought Volumes 5 and 6 of the third edition of Darwin's *Collected Works*, which contained *The Descent of Man*. Thirty years later, he counted this work among his ten "most significant books"(Freud, 1906, p. 245).

Darwin's book had caused a similar shock in Vienna as it had in Victorian England. But it was precisely for this reason that Freud thought it desirable that as many people as possible should learn that Darwin's theory had dealt the death blow to belief in God. However, Freud was well aware that Darwin himself was indifferent to religion and did not derive a clearly critical attitude towards religion from his theory. In a letter to the pastor and psychoanalyst Oskar Pfister, which deals with religion and psychoanalysis, Freud wrote:

> It is of course possible to take advantage of the human right to be irrational and go some way with analysis and then stop, rather on the pattern of Charles Darwin, who used to go regularly to church on Sundays.
>
> (Freud and Pfister 1963, p. 128)

Ch. Darwin's

gesammelte Werke.

Aus dem Englischen übersetzt

von

J. Victor Carus.

Autorisirte deutsche Ausgabe.

Fünfter Band.

Die Abstammung des Menschen. I. Band.

Mit sechsundzwanzig Holzschnitten.

STUTTGART.

E. Schweizerbart'sche Verlagshandlung (E. Koch).

1875.

Figure 1.9 Volume 5 of Darwin's *Collected Works*

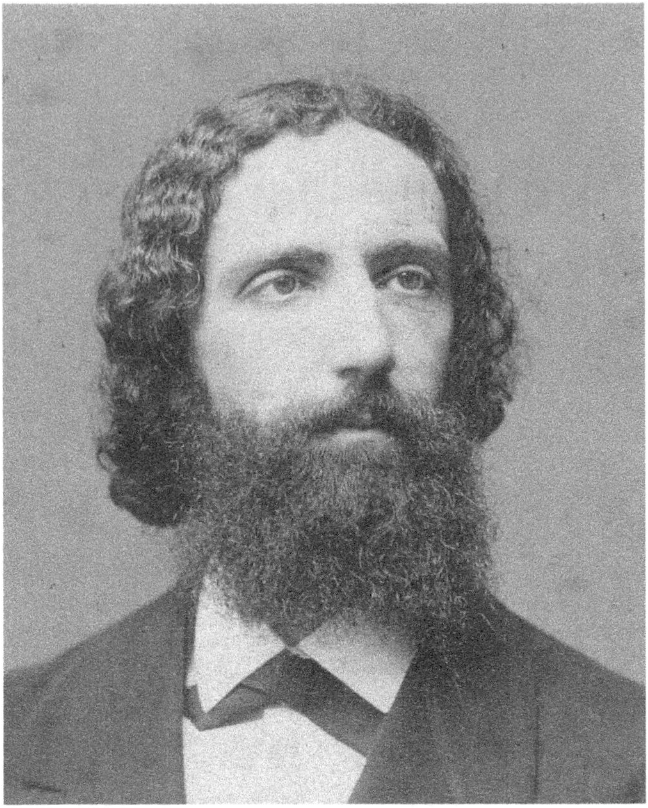

Figure 1.10 Franz Brentano, ca. 1875

However, not only zoologists taught at the University of Vienna, but also philosophers. One of them was Franz Brentano (1838–1917). He was a philosopher and psychologist, but had also studied theology and become a priest. Brentano publicly opposed the canonization of papal infallibility and criticized the dogmas of the Trinity and the Incarnation. In 1873, he renounced the priesthood and moved from the University of Würzburg to the University of Vienna. There, he was appointed Professor of Philosophy in 1874. In addition to attending lectures on zoology and natural history, Freud also attended Brentano's "In community with the students: Reading, explanation and critical discussion of selected philosophical writings," a colloquium on "The existence of God."

The "selected philosophical writings" included Ludwig Feuerbach's *The Essence of Christianity* and David Friedrich Strauss's *The Old and*

New Faith. Freud had written that he revered and admired Feuerbach "above all other philosophers" (Freud, 1990, p. 96) and that he had read him and Strauss "with pleasure and enthusiasm" (Freud and Binswanger, 2003, p. 179). John Stuart Mill's *The Principle of Utility* was also discussed. To "Mill's Thoughts" Freud hoped "to devote myself with zeal in the near future" (Freud, 1990, p. 97). Little did he know at the time that five years later he himself would be translating the 12th volume of Mill's *Collected Works* into German.

The colloquium "The Existence of God" provided the impetus for Freud's theoretical engagement with God, faith, and religion. In the spring of 1875, he and his friend and fellow student Josef Paneth wrote to Brentano and were invited by him and to his home and to take walks together. On these occasions, they mainly discussed the "existence of God." Freud could not escape Brentano's line of argument and admired his ability to defend theistic arguments without phrases and with great precision.

Freud was initially very taken with Brentano and wrote to his friend Eduard Silberstein about the colloquium on the "Existence of God":

> Prof. Brentano, who gives the lectures, is a splendid man, a scholar and philosopher, even though he deems it necessary to support this airy existence of God with his own expositions.
>
> (Freud, 1990, p. 71)

Under Brentano's influence, Freud even considered changing from the medical faculty to the philosophical faculty.

But Freud felt that it was only under Brentano's influence that he had become a theist of necessity. He saw this development as a consequence of his helplessness in the face of Brentano's arguments. After several weeks of intense discussion of the problem of the existence of God and Brentano's position, the philosopher finally ceased to interest Freud. As his friend Josef Paneth writes, they increasingly saw through Brentano's "way of constantly using words instead of concepts, of embarrassingly proving unimportant things and trying to sneak in important things, and of working with paralogisms (i.e., actually jokes)" (Paneth, 2007, S. 32).

But the 19-year-old Freud had developed a position on the problem of the existence of God, which he summarized as follows:

> . . . the existence of God cannot be settled by union debates, parliamentary speeches, or speculation, but only by logical and psychological studies, for which not everyone has a taste, no more so than for astronomical computations. Hence it is just as wrong to think everyone is competent to pronounce on the existence of God as on the existence of Neptune.
>
> (Freud, 1990, p. 111)

Here Freud's lifelong conviction that there is an "undeniable conflict" between religion and science begins to emerge.

1.2.5 "A very special religious effect on the abdominal organs"

At the beginning of Freud's second year of study – at the time of Freud's preoccupation with natural history and his disappointment with Brentano – Freud's first written criticism of religion is at first ironic, without theoretical argumentation.

It is found in a letter from Freud to his closest friend at the time, Eduard Silberstein. They had known each other since 1866, quickly became friends, learned Spanish together, founded an Academia Castellana, and wrote humorous texts. In their correspondence, which was partly conducted in Spanish, the two friends had given each other the names "Cipion" and "Berganza" in reference to Cervantes's conversations between dogs.

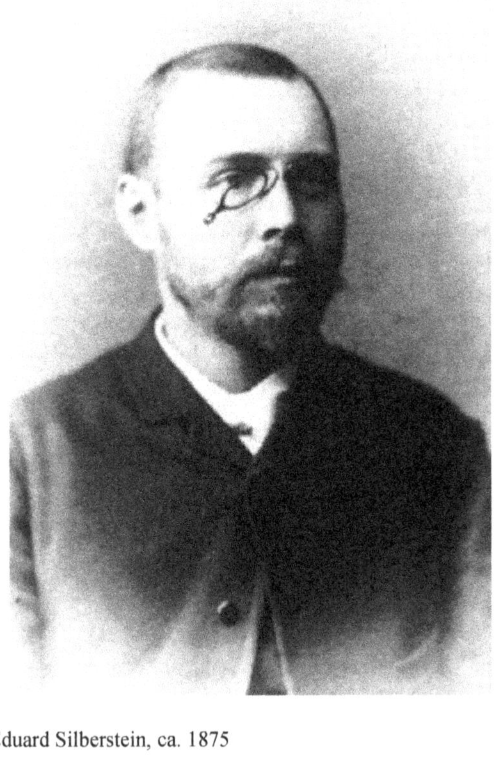

Figure 1.11 Eduard Silberstein, ca. 1875

Silberstein had now written that Freud might have forgotten the New Year, which in 1874 fell on 11 September, according to the Jewish calendar on the 29th of Elul. Freud replied on 18 September:

> To suggest that I might have overlooked the New Year is to impute to me a tastelessness of which I know myself to be completely free. People are wrong to reproach religion for being of a metaphysical nature and for lacking the certainty of sensory perceptions. Rather, religion addresses the senses alone, and even the Goddenier who is fortunate enough to belong to a tolerably pious family cannot deny the holiday when he puts a New Year's Day morsel to his lips. One might say that religion, consumed in moderation, stimulates the digestion, but that taken in excess it harms it. [. . .] Naturally enough, one's stomach is upset. It is most remarkable how certain holidays are distinguished by a very special religious effect on the abdominal organs. Thus the Passover has a constipating effect due to unleavened bread and hardboiled eggs. Yom Kippur is so lugubrious a day not so much through God's wrath as through the plum jam and the evacuation it stimulates.
>
> (Freud, 1990, p. 63)

This irony is also occasionally evident in Freud's letters over the next few years. For example, he ends a letter to Silberstein with the formula "praying that God's blessing be upon you, With cordial regards, Your Cipion" (Freud, 1990, p. 165). Or he wrote to his fiancée:

> It's such a holy Sunday silence, and the bells are ringing, I don't quite know why, and the streets are so clean, the people so polite, the old people look like I always imagined Christian Fürchtegott Gellert and the young are so modest, as if they already fear the good Lord.
>
> (Freud and Bernays, 2011, S. 205)

And even as late as 1925 he tried to offend an American visitor[6] by suggesting

> that the Statue of Liberty in New York harbor should be replaced by a monkey holding up a Bible.
>
> (Freud and Ferenczi, 2000, p. 227)

Probably Freud had read about the so-called Monkey Trial in Dayton, Tennessee, where a high school teacher, John Scopes, was accused of violating the Butler Act, a state law prohibiting the teaching of evolution in public schools. The trial became a national spectacle, pitting William Bryan, a fundamentalist hero, against Clarence Darrow, a renowned defense attorney, in a clash between science and religion.[7]

1.3 Engagement and wedding

1.3.1 Origin and family of the bride

In March 1882, one year after receiving his medical degree, Sigmund Freud met a 21-year-old young woman named Martha Bernays. She was visiting Freud's sisters with her sister Minna (Freud and Bernays, 2011, S. 32). On 17 June 1882, a few weeks after their first meeting, Sigmund and Martha became engaged.

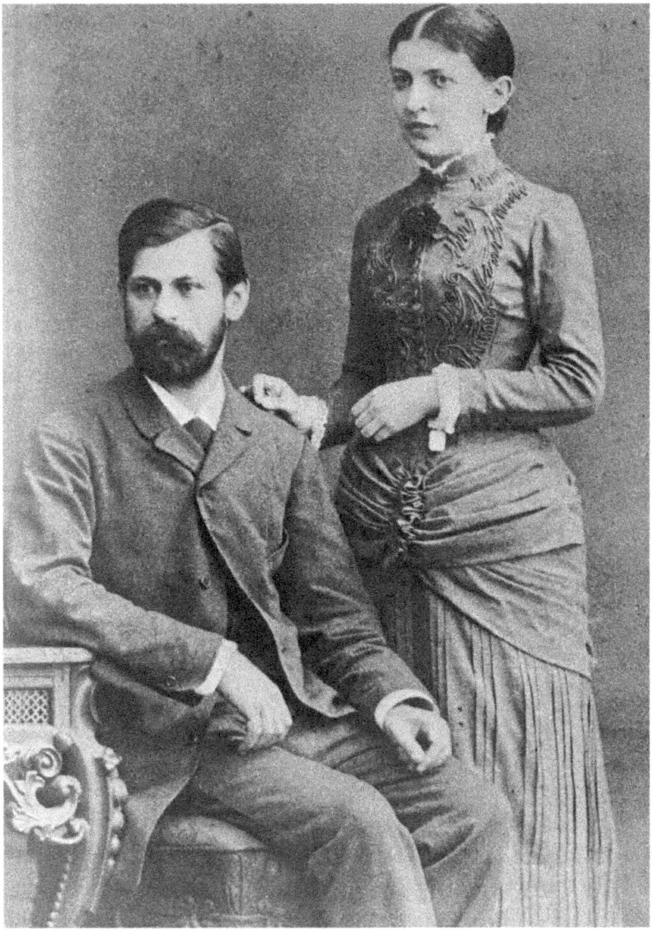

Figure 1.12 Freud with Martha Bernays, 1882

Martha was born in Hamburg and on 26 July 1861. Her paternal grandfather was Isaac Bernays (1792–1849), who was the Grand Rabbi of the German-Israelite community in Hamburg from 1821 until his death. He was one of the first to preach in German and was considered as a representative of modern Jewish Orthodoxy. His eldest son, Jacob Bernays (1824–1881), was a classical philologist and a friend of Theodor Mommsen. He was a committed Orthodox Jew and refused to convert to Christianity for professional reasons. His brother Michael Bernays (1834–1897) was quite different: he converted to Christianity as a young man. The middle son, Berman Bernays (1826–1879), was Martha's father.[8] He was a merchant, with only moderate success; he even had to serve a prison sentence for fraudulent bankruptcy. Not much more is known about his religious beliefs other than that he paid taxes to the Jewish community.

Less is known about Martha's maternal ancestors. Fabian Philipp (1756–1834), a brother of her great-grandfather, founded the first Jewish community in Karlskrona, Sweden, in 1785. He came from Bützow, only 40 km south of Rostock, and had arrived in Sweden in 1780. His nephew, Fabian Aaron (1790–1850), married Minna Ruben (1795–1861), who came from a highly respected Hamburg Jewish banking family. Her father Elias (1749–1822) was one of the co-founders and financial backers of the *Talmud Torah School* in Hamburg-Altona, founded in 1805 and the first strictly Jewish school in Hamburg. It quickly became the largest Jewish school in northern Germany. Around 1820, Minna Ruben and her husband Fabian Philipp moved from Karlskrona to Hamburg. Emmeline, Martha's mother, was born there in 1830. She died in 1910.

Thus, many members of Martha's mother's and father's families were, at least since the generation of their great-grandparents, firmly anchored in Jewish life in Northern Europe or actively involved in its development.

Martha's mother was opposed to the relationship and especially to a possible marriage, especially because of Freud's limited financial resources. This was one of the reasons why, two days after her secret engagement to Sigmund, she sent her daughter to Hamburg for three months, and in mid-June 1883 she moved there permanently with her daughters Martha and Minna to the north German port city. This meant that Martha and Sigmund were separated for almost four years between their engagement and their wedding on 13 September1886. During this time, the engaged couple exchanged some 1,600 letters and only saw each other only six times, mostly in secret, in Hamburg.

In the "Bridal Letters" from 1882 to 1886, "the face of the epoch is captured in many facets, but less in the sense of political events than of the history of mentality, the history of everyday life, the history of private life" (Freud and Bernays, 2011, S. 19). They also include Freud's occasional comments on Orthodox Jewish tradition and matters of faith.

1.3.2 "I was brought up without religion from the beginning": John Stuart Mill's autobiography

Freud was interested in the English philosopher John Stuart Mill (1806–1873) because he had read his writings at Brentano's colloquium. In 1879, possibly on Brentano's recommendation, he undertook the translation of the last volume of Theodor Gomperz's complete edition of the philosopher's works. Freud's translations were published in 1880 as volume 12 of Mill's *Gesammelte Werke* (Mill, 1880). Volume 12 contains the following writings by Mill: "On the Emancipation of Women"; "Plato"; "The Labor Question"; "Socialism."

In November 1883, Freud and his fiancée discussed Mill's ideas, especially those concerning the "emancipation of women."[9] It is noteworthy that Freud sent three pages from Mill's *Autobiography* to his bride, who came from an Orthodox Jewish rabbinical family in Hamburg and whose mother adhered to Orthodox traditions. He sent an excerpt of Mill's *Autobiography* to Martha with the note, "Recommended for reading to the little princess." Freud's excerpt begins with the sentence: "I was brought up [. . .] without any religious belief [. . .]" (Freud and Bernays, 2013, S. 459; cf. Mill, 1944, p. 27). It is remarkable that Freud used the same words some 40 years later in a letter

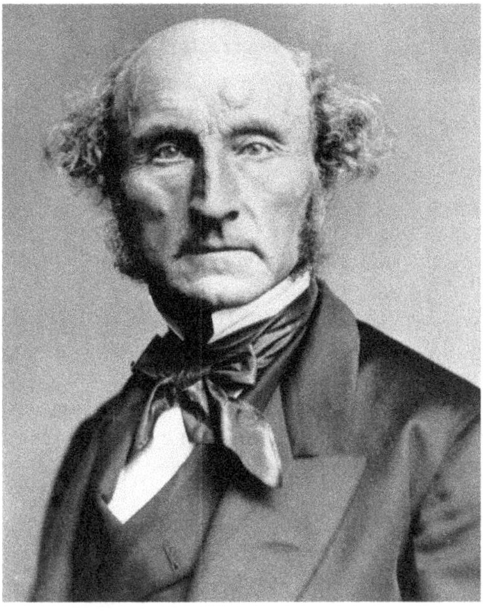

Figure 1.13 John Stuart Mill, ca. 1870

to the members of the Israelite Humanity Association B'nai B'rith on the occasion of his 70th birthday: "I [. . .] have been brought up without religion [. . .]" (Freud, 1961, S. 366).

The key sentences from the section of Mill's *Autobiography* Freud sent to Martha are:

> He[10] found it impossible to believe that a world so full of evil was the work of an Author combining infinite power with perfect goodness and righteousness. His intellect spurned the subtleties by which men attempt to blind themselves to this open contradiction. The Sabæan, or Manichæan theory of a Good and Evil Principle, struggling against each other for the government of the universe, he would not have equally condemned; and I have heard him express surprise, that no one revived it in our time. He would have regarded it as a mere hypothesis; but he would have ascribed to it no depraving influence. As it was, his aversion to religion, in the sense usually attached to the term, was of the same kind with that of Lucretius: he regarded it with the feelings due not to a mere mental delusion, but to a great moral evil. He looked upon it as the greatest enemy of morality: first, by setting up factitious excellencies, – belief in creeds, devotional feelings, and ceremonies, not connected with the good of human kind, – and causing these to be accepted as substitutes for genuine virtues: but above all, by radically vitiating the standard of morals; making it consist in doing the will of a being, on whom it lavishes indeed all the phrases of adulation, but whom in sober truth it depicts as eminently hateful. [. . .]
>
> This ne plus ultra of wickedness he considered to be embodied in what is commonly presented to mankind as the creed of Christianity. Think (he used to say) of a being who would make a Hell – who would create the human race with the infallible foreknowledge, and therefore with the intention, that the great majority of them were to be consigned to horrible and everlasting torment. The time, I believe, is drawing near when this dreadful conception of an object of worship will be no longer identified with Christianity; and when all persons, with any sense of moral good and evil, will look upon it with the same indignation with which my father regarded it. My father was as well aware as anyone that Christians do not, in general, undergo the demoralizing consequences which seem inherent in such a creed, in the manner or to the extent which might have been expected from it. The same slovenliness of thought, and subjection of the reason to fears, wishes, and affections, which enable them to accept a theory involving a contradiction in terms, prevents them from perceiving the logical consequences of the theory. Such is the facility with which mankind believe at one and the same time things inconsistent with one another, and so few are those who draw from what they receive as truths, any consequences but those recommended to them by their feelings, that multitudes have held the undoubting belief in an Omnipotent Author of

> Hell, and have nevertheless identified that being with the best conception they were able to form of perfect goodness. Their worship was not paid to the demon which such a being as they imagined would really be, but to their own idea of excellence. The evil is, that such a belief keeps the ideal wretchedly low; and opposes the most obstinate resistance to all thought which has a tendency to raise it higher. Believers shrink from every train of ideas which would lead the mind to a clear conception and an elevated standard of excellence, because they feel (even when they do not distinctly see) that such a standard would conflict with many of the dispensations of nature, and with much of what they are accustomed to consider as the Christian creed. And thus morality continues a matter of blind tradition, with no consistent principle, nor even any consistent feeling, to guide it.
>
> (Freud and Bernays, 2013, S. 460–462; cf. Mill, 1944, p. 28)

Surely Freud produced this translation not only to encourage his bride to adopt a more critical attitude toward religion, but also because it likely helped him to clarify his own positions.

1.3.3 The funeral of Nathan Weiss

Nathan Weiss (1851–1883) was a neurologist and the son of the Talmud teacher Isaak Weiss (1815–1905). Freud met him in 1883 at the Vienna

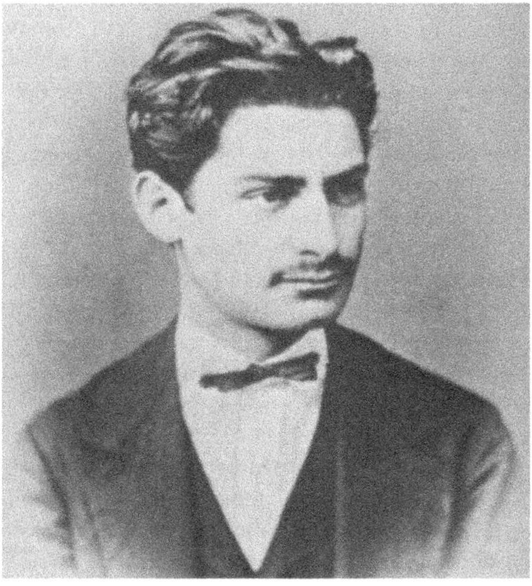

Figure 1.14 Nathan Weiss, ca. 1880

General Hospital, where Weiss had been working for five years and Freud had started as a secundarius aspirans. The two men became friends, and on 15 August 1883, Freud attended Nathan Weiss's wedding with Helene Strauss (1857–1921). A month later – shortly after returning from his honeymoon – Nathan hanged himself in a public bath in Vienna.

The funeral was held on 16 September. That same day, Freud wrote in a letter to his fiancée Martha:

> Families began to quarrel over his body, and a loud, discordant cry of vengeance rang out from his open grave, as unjust and pitiless as if he himself had uttered it. The scribe Friedmann, a relative and colleague of his old father, began: "Your name was Noah, and your parents attached the saying to it: 'You shall be my comfort and my support in my old age'; and all that comfort is here. And it is written: When a body is found, and it is not known by whose hand he died, then look ye to your neighbours, for they are the murderers. But we, his parents and brothers, did not shed his blood," and now he began to accuse the other family in clear words that they had given him the death blow. He spoke with the powerful voice of the fanatic, with the fervour of the savage, merciless Jew. We all froze with indignation and shame before the Christians among us. It was as if we had given them the right to believe that we worshiped the God of vengeance and not of love.
>
> (Freud and Bernays, 2013, S. 252)

Freud was embarrassed by the eulogist's words, and this experience may have contributed to the fact that Freud attended very few funerals in the half-century or so before his own death.

1.3.4 "Asking for cheese, after the meat dish": sabotage of Jewish holidays and violation of kosher dietary laws

On 10 September 1883, Freud's father had travelled to Manchester to visit his sons Emanuel and Philipp from his first marriage. He was expected back shortly after 2 October, which was the Jewish New Year that year. On 20 September, Freud wrote to his fiancée:

> The father should come soon after Rosh hash[11] Hammerschlag[12] has requested that I send my mother-in-law a letter of congratulations on this festive day; I have declared that I am at war with Judaism.
>
> (Freud and Bernays, 2013, S. 295)

And indeed, Freud did not write to his mother-in-law on the occasion of the New Year.

Freud was also familiar with the strict regulations of the Jewish religion for the preparation of food and drink. Those suitable for consumption are

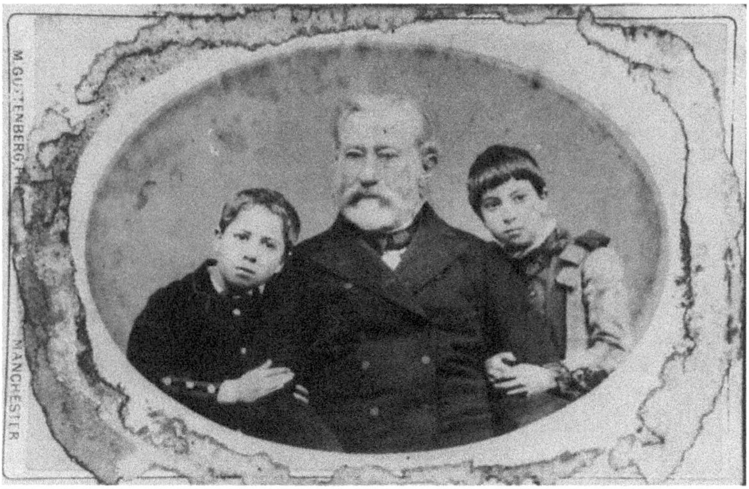

Figure 1.15 Jacob Freud with grandchildren Pauline and Morris, 1883

referred to as "kosher." One of the rules states that meaty and dairy foods may not be eaten at the same time and that a certain amount of time must pass after eating meaty foods before dairy foods may be eaten again. The Jewish dietary laws go back to the Torah and were later further specified.

An incident reported by Freud sheds light on his attitude to these rules: Freud spent March of 1886 in Berlin. There he spent time in various clinical institutions (cf. Toegel, 2006, S. 12–30). At the end of March, he received a visit from one of Martha's great cousins and her husband: Sally and Julius Lewisohn. Freud went with them to a performance of Kleist's play "Prince of Homburg" at the Deutsches Theater – incidentally with Josef Kainz in the leading role. Freud describes his impressions in a letter to Martha:

> The little theatre is small and wasn't full, a prologue spoken by a pink lady was horribly pompous and praised the old gentleman, who can no longer walk or stand, as "resplendent in full manhood". You know the play, the Lewisohns didn't, and I was able to follow the impression it made on them both. At first it was very disconcerting, the somnambulistic scene, which is really something strange in a Margravian colonel and war hero, was very astonishing. Sally went on to make a series of delicious remarks, such as: She would not like to marry the man, but she believed that if he were her husband she would drive the indecision out of him; how one could be so afraid of death, etc. But she understood very well the conflict that arose. He was even more decidedly unsatisfied. For him, as a merchant who is more interested in the end than the means, the question of whether or not

> one may win against the order was a settled one from the outset, and he said that a play that contained nothing else was boring. The many weaknesses of the play were actually quite noticeable to me too. . . .
>
> (Freud and Bernays, 2013, p. 355)

After the theatre, Freud went to dinner with his guests. He provoked the Jewish relatives by marriage with a "blunder": he committed the – probably intentional – faux pas of "asking for cheese after the meat dish" (Freud and Bernays, 2013, p. 356).

1.4 First years of marriage

A good two years before his own wedding, Freud attended the wedding of his closest friend Josef Paneth at the time, with Sophie Schwab on 15 May 1884. He wrote to his fiancée about the Jewish wedding ceremony:

> One room was turned into an exhibition, which I did not see, although it looked very pompous. [. . .] The wedding took place under a ridiculous canopy in a room that had been transformed into a temple-like wasteland. The priest, Jellinek, was very disgusting, though still relatively modest; he praised the parents, of course, and praised her to him, and him to her, as if they had been waiting for him to appreciate them, and he added the dear Lord God, who was to shower his very special favour on these two human children, and in between there was beautiful singing by the Chasan[13] in the moving tones of our old mother tongue. Breuer stood at the door and did not listen to the ghost; I was terribly annoyed at the whole barbarism, and that two good people should have to choke down religious hypocrisy at the moment when they were really moved and wanted to be more, and I thought how I could spare myself that, and came to Breuer with the project that I wanted to convert to Christianity, so that we would then have to enter into a civil marriage; but he rejected it as too complicated. Later I had the saving thought that we would probably get married in Wandsbek, where the civil ceremony must precede it, and that we could then dispense with the "church" ceremony altogether, and I resolved, if I still had enough strength at that time, to go through with it and to become very angry, perhaps even not to like you at all, if you insisted on the ritual marriage ceremony.
>
> (Freud and Bernays, 2015, S. 335–337)

Four months after his wedding, the bridegroom Josef Paneth wrote an essay entitled "Quid faciendum."[14] The essay is "in the intellectual world of those Jews [. . .] for whom the Jewish religion no longer means anything" (Paneth, 2007, S. 74). Paneth writes, among other things: "Judaism, in my eyes, is an anachronism. [. . .] It is a relic, a pet relic, long since worthy of extinction" (Paneth, 2007, S. 84).

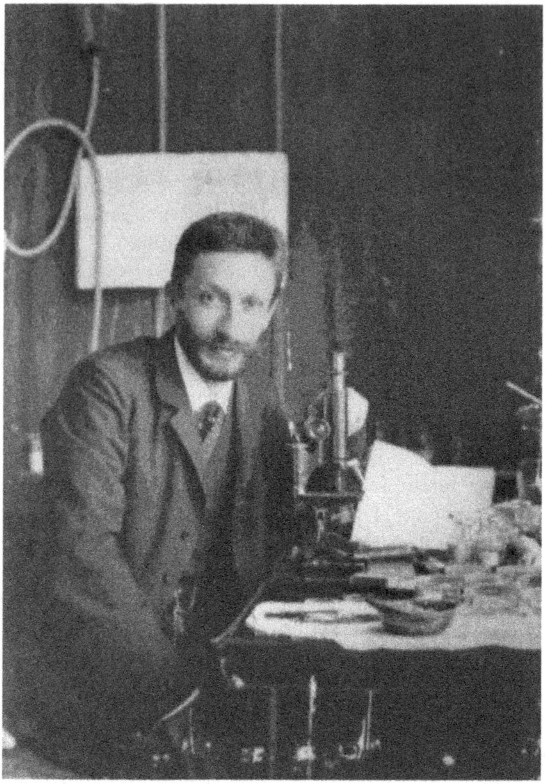

Figure 1.16 Josef Paneth, ca. 1880

Freud would have been familiar with the ideas in this essay. The two friends probably also discussed the basic ideas of the essay with each other. In any case, Freud's experiences and the ideas formulated in Paneth's essays had a direct impact on Freud's daily life and that of his family.

Only once did Freud participate in a religious ritual: his own Jewish wedding ceremony in Hamburg. Freud bowed only to Austrian law, which forced him to marry with a divine blessing. A civil marriage alone would not have been recognized in Austria. Freud made no further concessions.

On 13 September 1886, Sigmund and Martha's civil wedding took place at the Wandsbek Town Hall, and a day later the Jewish wedding took place at 32 Hamburgerstrasse, the home of Freud's mother-in-law. The lunch menu for the 12 wedding guests included fish salad, beef fillet, asparagus and peas, roast goose, and stewed fruit. The menu has survived, but no memory of the Jewish wedding ceremony.

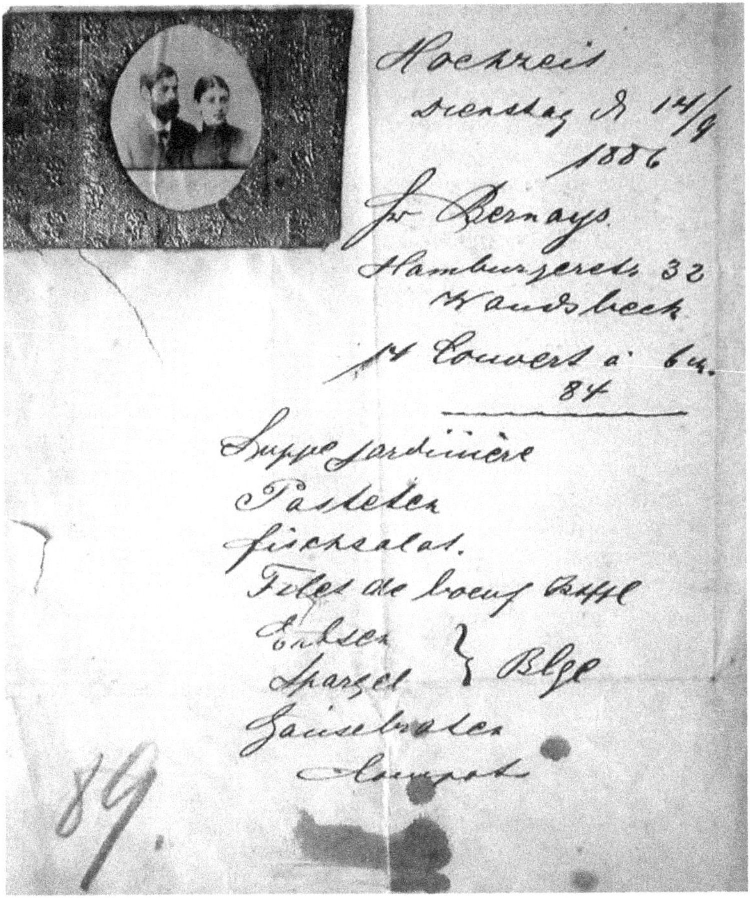

Figure 1.17 The wedding menu

The newlyweds set out on their honeymoon on the afternoon of 14 September, traveling via Lübeck, Travemünde, Berlin, Dresden, and Brno to Vienna. They arrived there on the evening of 29 September. They spent the night in a hotel because the lease on their apartment did not allow them to move in until the next day.

1.4.1 No lighting of the Sabbath candles

On 1 October 1886, a Friday, the couple moved into their apartment at 8 Maria-Theresien-Strasse. Martha was deeply saddened when she realized that her husband had not bought Sabbath candles. But she had known for some time that he detested religious rituals. Freud's attitude did not change throughout his life. An account of the Jewish catacombs in Rome, which he visited 20 years later on 21 September 1907, is indicative of this. In a postcard to Martha he writes,

> the [Jewish seven-branched] candelabrum can be seen on many tablets. Menorah, I think it's called. [. . .]
>
> (Freud, 2002, p. 223)

This comment too must have been painful for Martha.

1.4.2 No circumcision of the sons

Between 1887 and 1895, Martha had had six children, three of them sons: Martin (1889–1967), Oliver (1891–1969), and Ernst (1892–1970). The Jewish community birth records list all three sons as uncircumcised (see Figures 19, 20, and 21).

In Freud's writings and letters from these years there is no statement by Freud on the ritual of circumcision. But a year before his death, in his posthumously published *An Outline of Psycho-Analysis*, he formulated his view on the subject in a single sentence:

> The primaeval custom of circumcision, another symbolic substitute for castration, can only be understood as an expression of submission to the father's will.
>
> (Freud, 1940, p. 190)

1.4.3 The family Bible and Freud's alleged knowledge of Hebrew

To celebrate Freud's 35th birthday, his father gave him the family Bible. Published in 1839 by Ludwig Philippson, it was edited in Hebrew and German.

The Bible contains two inscriptions by Freud's father, Jacob, written in Hebrew on a commemorative page. One records the death of his father, Schlomo; the other, the birth of his son, Sigmund:

> My son Shlomo Sigismund, may he live, was born on Tuesday, Rosh Hodesh Iyar [5]616, 6:30 P.M., on May 6, [1]856 and was circumcised on Tuesday, the 8th day of the month of Iyar, on May 13, [1]856. The mohel [circumciser] was Reb Shimshon Frankel of Ostrau [Moravska Ostrava], godparents were Reb Lippe and his sister Mirel Hurwitz, children of the rabbi of Czernowitz. The sandek [the man who holds the infant on his knees during the circumcision] was Reb Shmuel Samueli.
>
> (Aron, 1956–57, p. 44)

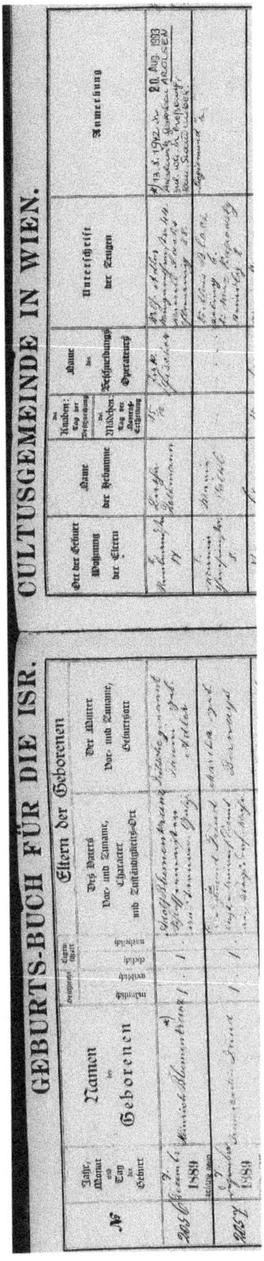
GEBURTS-BUCH FÜR DIE ISR. CULTUSGEMEINDE IN WIEN.

№	Jahr, Monat und Tag der Geburt	Namen der Geborenen	Eltern der Geborenen: Des Vaters Vor- und Zuname, Charakter und Zuständigkeits-Ort	Eltern der Geborenen: Der Mutter Vor- und Zuname, Geburtsort	Ort der Geburt, Wohnung der Eltern	Name der Hebamme	Name des Beschneiders, Operateurs	Unterschrift der Zeugen	Anmerkung
9056	1889	[illegible]	[illegible]	[illegible]	[illegible]	[illegible]	[illegible]	[illegible]	[illegible] 20. Aug. 1993 AROLSEN
9057	1889	[illegible]	[illegible]	[illegible]	[illegible]	[illegible]	[illegible]	[illegible]	[illegible]

Figure 1.18 Birth entry of Martin Freud

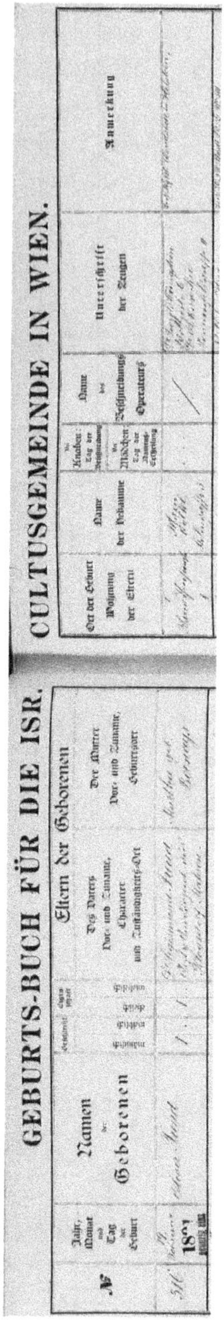

GEBURTS-BUCH FÜR DIE ISR. CULTUSGEMEINDE IN WIEN.

№	Jahr, Monat und Tag der Geburt	Namen der Geborenen	Geschlecht	Eltern der Geborenen: Des Vaters Vor- und Zuname, Charakter und Zuständigkeits-Ort	Der Mutter Vor- und Zuname, Geburtsort	Ort der Geburt, Wohnung der Eltern	Name der Hebamme	Name des Beschneidungs-Operateurs	Unterschrift der Zeugen	Anmerkung
516	1891	Oliver Freud	[illegible]	[illegible]	[illegible]	[illegible]	[illegible]	[illegible]	[illegible]	[illegible]

Figure 1.19 Birth entry of Oliver Freud

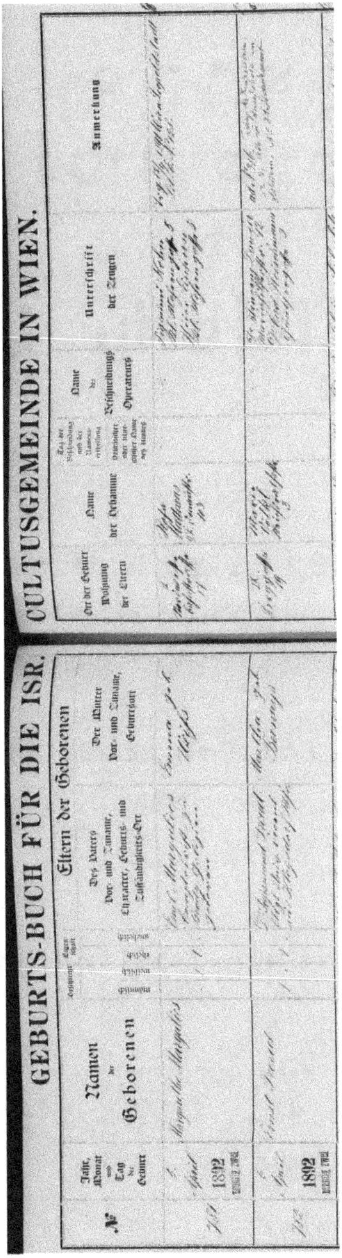

Figure 1.20 Birth entry of Ernst Freud

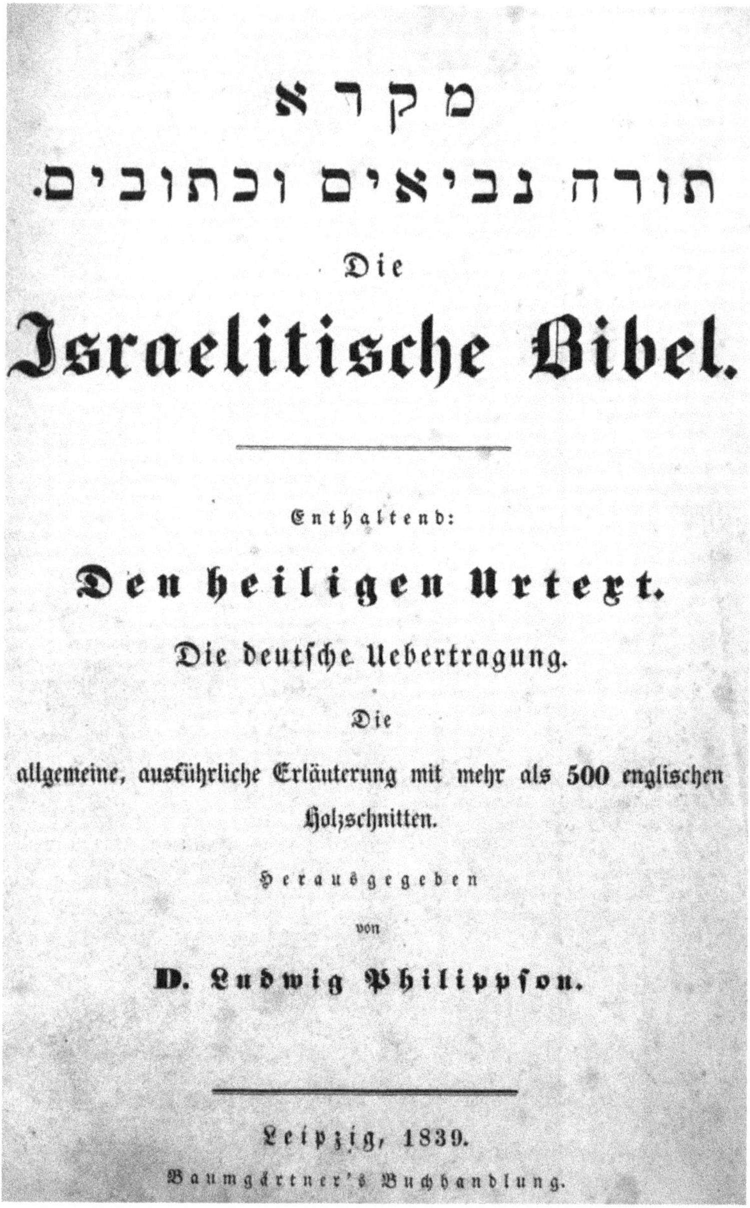

מקרא

תורה נביאים וכתובים.

Die

Israelitische Bibel.

Enthaltend:

Den heiligen Urtext.

Die deutsche Uebertragung.

Die

allgemeine, ausführliche Erläuterung mit mehr als 500 englischen Holzschnitten.

Herausgegeben

von

D. Ludwig Philippson.

Leipzig, 1839.

Baumgärtner's Buchhandlung.

Figure 1.21 The "Philippson Bible"

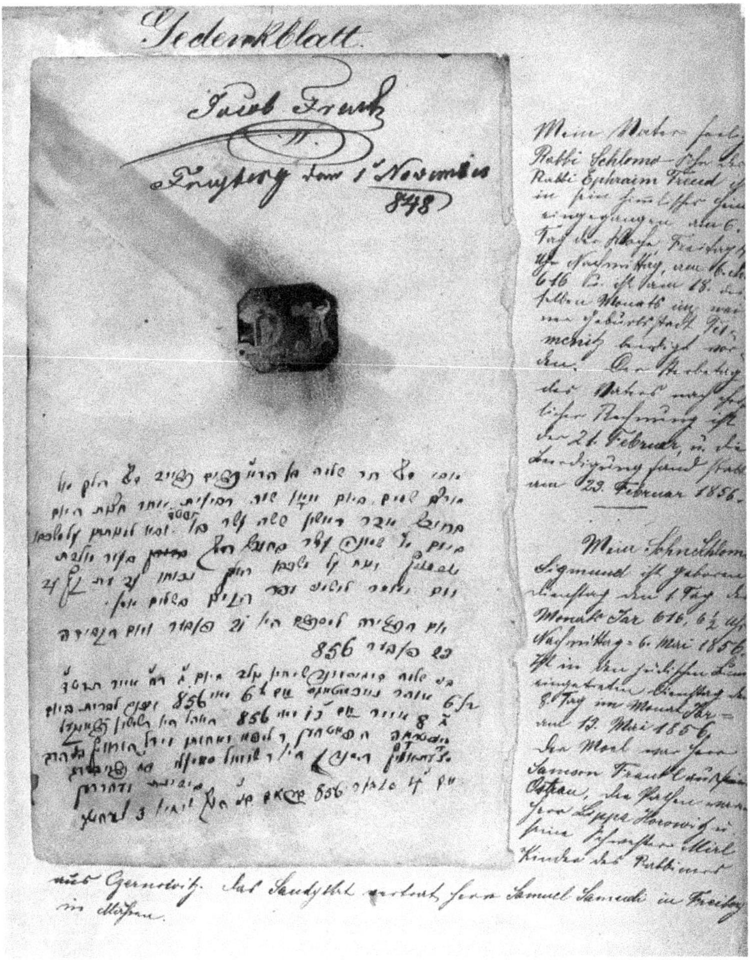

Figure 1.22 The commemorative page

The third inscription, also in Hebrew, was made on the occasion of Sigmund's 35th birthday. Jacob presented the family Bible to his eldest son, Sigmund, with the following dedication:

My Darling Son Shlomo
At the age of seven the spirit of the Lord began to move you
And spoke to you: Go read the books I have written

And there will break open to you the fountains of wisdom, knowledge and understanding.
The Book of Books is the well that the sages digged
And [in which] the lawgivers taught knowledge and justice.
The vision of the Almighty you saw, you heard, and you ventured,
You ascended and rode upon the wings of the spirit.
From then on that book was hidden like the Broken Tablets
In an Ark with me.
On the day you attained your thirty-fifth birthday
I bound it in a new leather binding
And named it "Spring up, O well – sing ye unto it"
And dedicated it to your name and for a remembrance of love.
From your father, who loves you an eternal love
Jacob son of Rabbi Shlomo Freud
In the capital city of Vienna, on the 29th of Nisan [5]651, May 6, [1]891.

(Aron, 1956–57, p. 44)

Years later, the commemorative entries were translated into German and the dedication into English. These translations were added to the family Bible. This was obviously necessary because Sigmund could not read or understand Hebrew. It is worth quoting some of Freud's statements to prove this.

The weekly newspaper *Jüdische Presszentrale Zürich*, founded in 1918 by Oscar Grün (1890–1953), began publishing a series entitled "Jewish Personalities in the Past and Present" in 1925. The first person to be featured was Moses Maimonides, followed by Arthur Schnitzler. The third was Sigmund Freud. In this context, Oscar Grün had asked Freud to provide him with information about his relationship with Judaism. On 1 January 1925 Freud answered:

> In the time of my youth our free-thinking religious instructors set no store by their pupils' acquiring a knowledge of the Hebrew language and literature. My education in this field was therefore extremely behindhand, as I have since often regretted.
>
> (Freud, 1925b, Feb., p. 291)

Three years later, in September 1928, Freud received the Hebrew translation of *Group Psychology and the Analysis of the Ego* from Hitachdut Hamorim Ha-Jehudim Erez Israel (the Association of Hebrew Teachers). On 9 September 1928, he responded:

> It is with particular satisfaction that I have taken up the translation of my Group Psychology into our sacred language. As an ignorant child of a pre-Zionist era, I am unfortunately unable to read it, but I am delighted by your

> assurance that this translation will serve an audience to whom the existing German or English editions would have meant nothing.
>
> (FML)

The Bible teacher Yehuda Dvir-Dvosis (1896–1971), who had already translated Freud's *Group Psychology and the Analysis of the Ego* into Hebrew in 1927, has asked Freud in the fall of 1930 if he would write prefaces for the Hebrew translations of the *Introductory Lectures* and *Totem and Taboo*. In his answering letter Freud wrote:

> It gives me extraordinary pleasure and satisfaction that some of my books will appear in the Hebrew language. My father spoke the holy language as well as German or even better. He let me grow up in perfect ignorance on everything concerning Judaism.
>
> (Rice, 1990, p. 44)

And eight years later, after receiving the proofs of the Hebrew translation of *Totem and Taboo* he wrote to Dvir-Dvosis:

> I am very pleased to hear that the Hebrew edition ofTotem and Taboo is about to appear. Since then I have also received a parcel which I believe are the proofs of the book (I, unfortunately, cannot read Hebrew).
>
> (Rice, 1990, p. 44)

Clearly, Freud could not read Hebrew, let alone understand it.

Notes

1 Kurt Eissler's interview with Hella Bernays, p. 15 (SFP).
2 *Jahresbericht des Lesevereines deutscher Studenten Wien's über das IV. Vereinsjahr 1874–75*. Wien. Selbstverlag des Lesevereines der deutschen Studenten, p. 3.
3 Only the building in Schönlaterngasse still stands today, see Figure 8, on the far right.
4 Cf. on the problem in more detail Hellige, H.-D. (1979). Generationenkonflikt, Selbsthaß und die Entstehung antikapitalistischer Positionen im Judentum. Der Einfluß des Antisemitismus auf das Sozialverhalten jüdischer Kaufmanns-und Unternehmersöhne im Deutschen Kaiserreich und in der K.u.K.-Monarchie. *Geschichte und Gesellschaft*, *5*, 476–518.
5 *Das Freie Blatt*, 5.11.1872, p. 2.
6 Presumably George Davis Bivin (1874–1934).
7 Thanks to Ernst Falzeder.
8 The information about Martha's family comes mainly from the following sources: Behling, K. (2002). *Martha Freud. Die Frau des Genies*. Berlin: Aufbau Taschenbuch Verlag; Brämer, A. (2000). *Judentum und*

religiöse Reform. Der Hamburger Israelitische Tempel 1817–1938. Hamburg: Dölling und Gallitz Verlag; Brämer, A. (2006). Isaak Bernays. In K. Heinsohn (Ed.), *Das Jüdische Hamburg. Ein historisches Nachschlagewerk.* Wallstein Verlag; Hirschmüller, A. (2005). Zur Familie Bernays. In A. Hirschmüller (Ed.), *Sigmund Freud – Minna Bernays. Briefwechsel 1882–1938.* Edition Diskord, S. 325–343; Randt, U. (1991). Jüdische Schulen am Grindel. In U. Wamser & W. Weinke (Eds.), *Ehemals in Hamburg zu Hause. Jüdisches Leben am Grindel.* VSA-Verlag, S. 36–55; Singer, I., & Sohn, J. (1902). Michael Bernays. In I. Singer (Ed.), *The Jewish Encyclopedia.* Funk and Wagnall, Vol. 3., S. 92f; Valentin, H. (1924). *Judarnas Historia i Sverige.* Stockholm: Bonnier, 224f; Wolff, W., & Wolff, M. (2014). *Das eigene Leben erzählen. Geschichte und Biografie von Hamburger Juden aus zwei Generationen.* Hg. von Linde Apel. Göttingen: Wallstein.

9 Freud, S., & Bernays, M. (2013). *Die Brautbriefe.* Band 2. Unser "Roman in Fortsetzungen." Juli 1883–Dezember 1883. Ed. by Gerhard Fichtner, Ilse Grubrich-Simitis und Albrecht Hirschmüller. Frankfurt am Main: S. Fischer, 424f.

10 Mill's father.

11 The editors of the *Brautbriefe* probably correctly assume that "Rosh hash" is an ironic reference to the Jewish New Year's holiday of "Rosh Hashanah" (Freud, S., & Bernays, M. (2013). *Die Brautbriefe.* Band 2. Unser "Roman in Fortsetzungen." Juli 1883–Dezember 1883. Ed. by Gerhard Fichtner, Ilse Grubrich-Simitis und Albrecht Hirschmüller. Frankfurt am Main: S. Fischer, S. 297).

12 Freud's religious teacher Samuel Hammerschlag (1826–1904), with whose family Freud was on friendly terms.

13 Cantor of the synagogue.

14 "What to do."

2 Critique of religion in Freud's writings

Between 1907 and 1939 Freud published several writings critical of religion. They were and are the subject of numerous publications, including by representatives of various religions. These will not be discussed here. Instead, only Freud's core ideas on religion are summarized as follows.

2.1 "Religion as a universal obsessional neurosis" (1907)

After Freud's preoccupation with Mill's description of his and his father's conception of religion in 1883, it would be more than 20 years before Freud would again write on questions of religion. This time, however, it was a scientific approach.

In early 1907, Johannes Bresler, the editor of the *Psychiatrisch-Neurologische Wochenschrift*, asked Freud to become co-editor of the new *Zeitschrift für Religionspsychologie* that he had founded. Freud accepted and wrote an article for the first issue entitled "Obsessive Actions and Religious Practices." The article begins with the following statement:

> I am certainly not the first person to have been struck by the resemblance between what are called obsessive actions in sufferers from nervous affections and the observances by means of which believers give expression to their piety. The term "ceremonial", which has been applied to some of these obsessive actions, is evidence of this. The resemblance, however, seems to me to be more than a superficial one, so that an insight into the origin of neurotic ceremonials may embolden us to draw inferences by analogy about the psychological processes of religious life.
>
> (Freud, 1907, p. 117)

What compulsive acts and religious rituals have in common is the guilty conscience that results from failure to act. In this respect, compulsive neurosis is a "half funny, half sad" private religion. The motives underlying the religious practice are unknown to the believers or are represented in their consciousness

DOI: 10.4324/9781003674047-2

by pretended motives. According to Freud, the obsessive-compulsive patient is under the influence of a guilt feeling of which he is unaware. This corresponds to the believer's self-image of actually being a sinner. The religious ritual is a kind of defense or protection against this. In addition, compulsive acts and religious practices share the fact that they are based on the renunciation of certain impulses: in neurosis, these are usually sexual impulses; in religion, they are more likely to be selfish or socially harmful impulses, usually with a sexual component as well. The renunciation of impulses in religion is intended to prevent divine punishment. Relapse, that is, unsuccessful renunciation of urges, leads to new religious activities – acts of penance as self-punishment.

For Freud, obsessional neurosis is the pathological counterpart of religious practice; that is, he sees neurosis as an individual religion and "religion as a universal obsessional neurosis" (Freud, 1907, p. 126).

2.2 The "final cause of religions": infantile helplessness (1910)

In his essay "Obsessive Actions and Religious Practices" Freud deals only with analogous mechanisms, not with causal connections. Freud first referred to these on 27 October 1909 at the Vienna Psychoanalytic Society: In the discussion of Fritz Wittels' "Analysis of a Hysterical State of Confusion," he remarked,

> This case also shows distinctly in what way religious instruction acts upon the lives of Catholic children. How many a germ of psychosis enter the child's brain along this path! The Christ-fantasy that is clearly present in this case also goes back to that.
>
> (Nunberg and Federn, 1967, vol. 2, p. 285)

Just a few weeks later, Freud believed he had discovered the "ultimate reason for religions." He wrote to Carl Gustav Jung on 2 January 1910:

> Of my own flashes of inspiration [. . .] I can confide only one. It has occurred to me that the ultimate basis of man's need for religion is infantile helplessness, which is so much greater in man than in animals. After infancy he cannot conceive of a world without parents and makes for himself a just God and a kindly nature, the two worst anthropomorphic falsifications he could have imagined.
>
> (Freud and Jung, 1974, p. 282)

Helplessness in the face of death was the main reason why people created evil spirits, which proved to be the precursors of mythological beings and religious deities (Freud, 1913).

2.3 "Magic and the omnipotence of thoughts" (1913)

In his book *Totem and Taboo*, published in 1913, Freud took up the basic idea of the 1907 article on "Compulsive Acts and Religious Practice." Here he developed his ideas about the similarity between religion and the customs

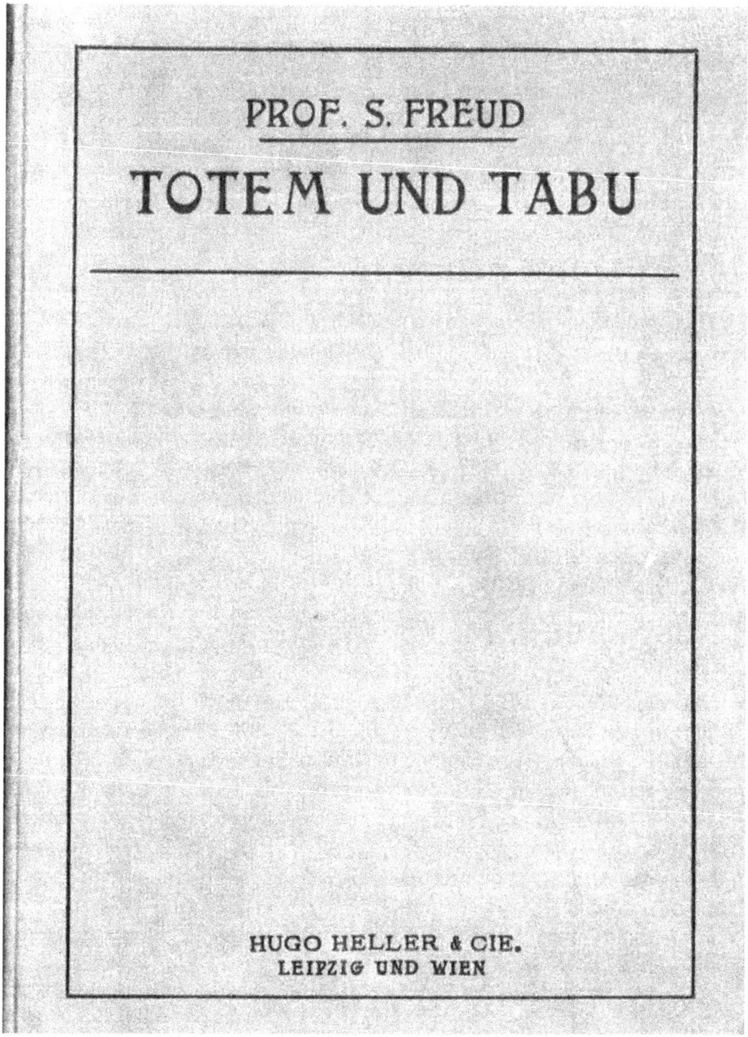

Figure 2.1 The cover of *Totem and Taboo*

of "primitive" peoples and the unconscious fantasies of his neurotic patients. The subtitle formulates the work's concern in language that hardly any publisher today would accept: "Some Points of Agreement Between the Mental Lives of Savages and Neurotics."

Freud had begun writing in the spring of 1911, but after six months the work came to a standstill, as he confessed to Carl Gustav Jung: "In my work on totemism I have run into all sorts of difficulties, rapids, waterfalls, sandbanks, etc.; I don't know yet if I shall be able to float my craft again" (Freud and Jung, 1974, p. 468). And a little later he confesses to his Hungarian colleague Sándor Ferenczi:

> The work on totem is a mess. I am reading fat books without any real interest, since I know the conclusions already; my instinct tells me so. But all the material has to be ground through, and in the meantime the insights become clouded. There are many things that don't want to make sense, and yet shouldn't be forced, and I don't have time every evening, etc. Sometimes I feel as though I only wanted to start a little liaison and at my age discovered that I had to marry a new wife.
>
> (Freud and Ferenczi, 1993, p. 316)

Although the work on this work was anything but easy for him, Freud had the "feeling that it is my greatest, best, and perhaps my last good thing" (Freud and Ferenczi, 1993, p. 482). *Totem and Taboo* was completed on 12 May 1913, and on 29 June Freud celebrated its publication with friends and followers at a restaurant on the Konstantinshügel in Vienna's Prater with a "Totem Festival."

The first section deals with "The Horror of Incest" and the second section with "Taboo and Emotional Ambivalence." It is only in the third section, entitled "Animism, Magic and the Omnipotence of Thoughts," that the origin of religion is finally discussed. Animism is a stage of human development in which the world is populated by souls and demons, and people project some of their desires onto the spirits around them. Freud distinguishes magic as a technique for influencing other people, especially enemies, and the outside world from sorcery – methods for bringing spirits under control. One of the most common magical procedures is to create an image of an enemy from any material. Whatever is done to the image is done to the hated enemy. Or you can magically create rain by imitating it or the clouds that produce it.

For Freud, however, the real essence of magic is the "omnipotence of thought," the exaggerated belief in the power of wishes, as seen in the fantasies of neurotics and the wishes of children. Above all, the confrontation with the experience of death is the reason why man invented evil spirits, which turned out to be the forerunners of mythological beings and religious deities. Alluding to magic and the "omnipotence of thought,"

Freud wrote in his letter of congratulations on Thomas Mann's 60th birthday:

> I am one of your oldest readers and admirers. I should wish you a long and happy life, as is customary on such occasions. But I refrain from doing so; wishing is cheap, and it seems to me a throwback to the days when people believed in the magical omnipotence of thought.
>
> (Wysling, 1988, p. 186)

In the fourth and longest section, "The Return of Totemism in Childhood," Freud sums up the view that

> totemism is a system which takes the place of a religion among certain primitive peoples of Australia, America and Africa, and provides the basis of their social organization.
>
> (Freud, 1913, p. 100)

Freud also points out an exception: the sacrificial meal. By sacrificing and eating the totem animal together, which is actually taboo, the relationship between the clan members is strengthened. The sons who killed their father repeat the patricide with every sacrificial ceremony. In this way, the community is strengthened and maintained not only among the brothers, but also with the forefather, whose powers they acquire by eating him and repeating them in the sacrificial meal. Freud sees the totem meal as a repetition of patricide and

> a commemoration of this memorable and criminal deed, which was the beginning of so many things – of social organization, of moral restrictions and of religion.
>
> (Freud, 1913, p. 142)

In the year *Totem and Taboo* was published, Freud was visited by Ludwig Binswanger and Paul Häberlin. The latter recalled a conversation: "For him there was no norm. What seemed to be the norm was transformed neediness, transformed libido, parental influence accepted out of a desire to conform to the parents. Religion was a priestly invention, even a priestly deception.[1]

2.4 Sophocles and Euripides: "Legendary material an indictment of the gods and fate [. . .]" (1916)

Freud had announced *Introductory lectures on Psycho-Analysis* for the winter semester of 1914/15, but did not give them (Gicklhorn and Gicklhorn, 1960, pp. 155, 191). The first of these lectures did not take place until a year later, on 23 October 1915, and Freud wrote about it to Sándor Ferenczi on 31 October:

> My mornings are almost completely free. In all this leisure I have decided to inaugurate the lectures, and on October 23 and 30 I found myself facing a college of about seventy persons, among them two daughters and a daughter-in-law.[2] So it was incumbent upon to me to make more out of the lecture than usual, to prepare myself properly, and as things continued I arrived at the intention also to publish the lectures I gave this way.
>
> (Freud and Ferenczi, 1996, p. 85)

By the fourth lecture the audience had grown to 100 and Freud gradually began to write up his lectures. On 1 January 1916 the manuscript of the first four lectures was expected by the publisher Heller, who wanted to publish them in February. However, due to the war, printing was delayed until 10 July (Freud and Andreas-Salomé, 1963, p. 47). The second part with *Lectures* 5 to 15 appeared in mid-December 1916, the third part in early June 1917, and the reprint in one volume in mid-June.

The 21st *Lecture* is entitled "The Development of the Libido and the Sexual Organizations." In this lecture, Freud also introduces his audience to the Oedipus complex. He begins with a true story:

> Listen to this episode which occurred in the course of the present war. One of the stout disciples of psycho-analysis was stationed as medical officer on the German front somewhere in Poland. He attracted his colleagues' attention by the fact that he occasionally exercised an unexpected influence on a patient. When he was questioned, he acknowledged that he was employing the methods of psycho-analysis and declared his readiness to convey his knowledge to his colleagues. Every evening there after the medical officers of the corps, his colleagues and his superiors, came together in order to learn the secret doctrines of analysis. All went well for a while; but when he spoke to his audience about the Oedipus complex, one of his superiors rose, declared he did not believe it, that it was a vile act on the part of the lecturer to speak of such things to them, honest men who were fighting for their country and fathers of a family, and that he forbade the continuance of the lectures. That was the end of the matter. The analyst got himself transferred to another part of the front. It seems to me a bad thing, however, if a German victory requires that science shall be "organized" in this way, and German science will not respond well to organization of such a kind.
>
> And now you will be eager to hear what this terrible Oedipus complex contains. Its name tells you. You all know the Greek legend of King Oedipus, who was destined by fate to kill his father and take his mother to wife,

> who did everything possible to escape the oracle's decree and punished himself by blinding when he learned that he had none the less unwittingly committed both these crimes. I hope many of you may yourselves have felt the shattering effect of the tragedy in which Sophocles has treated the story. The work of the Athenian dramatist exhibits the way in which the long-past deed of Oedipus is gradually brought to light by an investigation ingeniously protracted and fanned into life by ever fresh relays of evidence. To this extent it has a certain resemblance to the progress of a psycho-analysis. In the course of the dialogue Jocasta, the deluded mother and wife, declares herself opposed to the continuance of the enquiry. She appeals to the fact that many people have dreamt of lying with their mothers, but that dreams should be despised. We do not despise dreams – least of all, typical dreams which occur to many people; and we do not doubt that the dream referred to by Jocasta has an intimate connection with the strange and terrifying content of the legend.
>
> It is a surprising thing that the tragedy of Sophocles does not call up indignant repudiation in his audience – a reaction similar to that of our simple-minded army doctor but far better justified. For fundamentally it is an amoral work: it absolves men from moral responsibility, exhibits the gods as promoters of crime and shows the impotence of the moral impulses of men which struggle against crime. It might easily be supposed that the material of the legend had in view an indictment of the gods and of fate; and in the hands of Euripides, the critic and enemy of the gods, it would probably have become such an indictment. But with the devout Sophocles there is no question of an application of that kind. The difficulty is overcome by the pious sophistry that to bow to the will of the gods is the highest morality even when it promotes crime. I cannot think that this morality is a strong point of the play, but it has no influence on its effect.
>
> (Freud, 1917, p. 330)

There is no doubt that Freud here disagrees with Sophocles, but accuses him of "pious sophistry" and suspects that under Euripides's pen the tragedy would have turned into an indictment of the gods. Freud certainly knew that Euripides had also worked the Oedipus material into a tragedy, but that it was lost. Freud also knew that Euripides's criticism of religion made him the object of intense hostility, a fate that Freud could not escape.

2.5 Preface to Theodor Reik's *Psychology of Religion* (1919)

Theodor Reik (1888–1969) studied philosophy and literature in Vienna. He wrote his doctoral thesis on "The psychogenesis of Flaubert's 'The Temptation of St. Anthony'. A contribution to the psychology of artists." It was published as a book with a preface by the famous journalist and

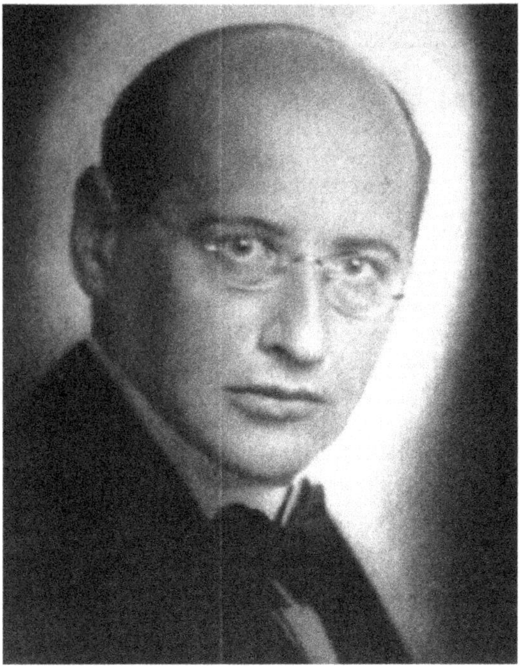

Figure 2.2 Theodor Reik, ca. 1925

theatre critic Alfred Kerr (Reik, 1912). Reik had visited Freud in 1910, who advised him to devote himself to psychoanalytic studies (Mühlleitner, 1992, p. 260). In November 1911, Reik became a member of the Vienna Psychoanalytical Society. In 1918, at Freud's suggestion, his work *Die Pubertätsriten der Wilden* (Reik, 1915/1916) was awarded the prize of the journal *Imago for* the best scientific work in the field of applied psychoanalysis. His treatise book *Ritual: Psycho-Analytic Studies* (*Probleme der Religionspsychologie*) was published as Volume 5 of the International Psychoanalytic Library.

In his preface to the book, Freud writes:

> If one subjects the prehistoric and ethnological material [. . .] to a psychoanalytical treatment, an unexpectedly precise result emerges: that God the Father once walked the earth in the flesh and, as chieftain of the primitive human horde, used his ruling power until his sons slew him in unison. Furthermore, that through the effect of this liberating atrocity and in reaction

> to it, the first social bonds came into being, the basic moral restrictions and the oldest form of religion, totemism. But that the later religions are also filled with the same content and endeavor, on the one hand, to cover up the traces of that crime or to atone for it by using other solutions for the struggle between father and sons, but on the other hand cannot avoid repeating the elimination of the father anew. The echoes of that event, which overshadowed the entire development of humanity, can also be recognized in the myth.
>
> This hypothesis, which is founded on the observations of Robertson Smith and was developed by me in *Totem and Taboo*, has been taken by Theodor Reik as the basis of his studies on the problems of the psychology of religion, of which this is the first volume. In accordance with psycho-analytic technique these studies start out from hitherto unexplained details of religious life, and by means of their elucidation gain access to the fundamental postulates and ultimate aims of religions; moreover they keep steadily in view the relation between prehistoric man and contemporary primitive societies as well as the connection between the products of civilization and the substitutive structures of neurotics.
>
> (Freud, 1919, p. 262)

Almost ten years later, Freud himself was to devote himself to the "elucidation of the deepest preconditions [. . .] and ultimate goals of religions." His main work critical of religion, *The Future of an Illusion*, also deals with this question.

2.6 *The Future of an Illusion* (1927)

In the spring of 1927 Freud began work on his book *The Future of an Illusion*. He had long delayed writing it down and publishing his thoughts out of respect for his friend Pastor Oskar Pfister. In contrast to his earlier works on the subject, the book is primarily concerned with the nature and future of religion. Freud emphasized the distinction that an illusion is not an error, but a belief that is essentially motivated by wish fulfilment – for example, when a poor girl indulges in the illusion that a prince will come and marry her. Freud was aware that his theories would meet with strong opposition, but he knew how to console himself:

> In former times it was different. Then utterances such as mine brought with them a sure curtailment of one's earthly existence and an effective speeding-up of the opportunity for gaining a personal experience of the after-life.
>
> (Freud, 1927, p. 36)

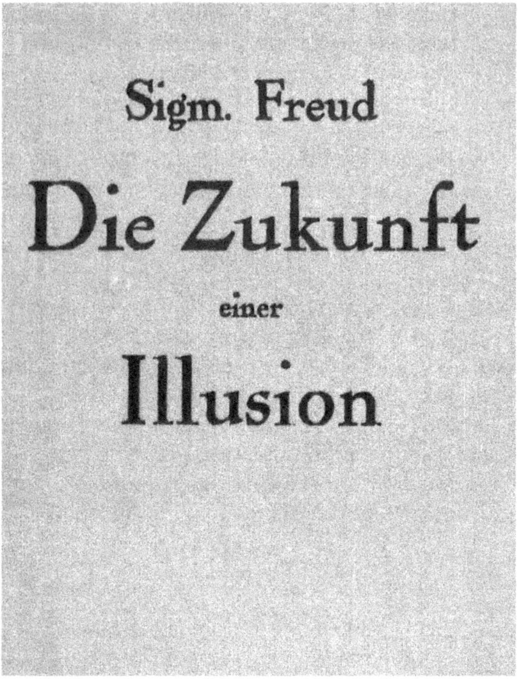

Figure 2.3 The cover of *The Future of an Illusion*

In line with his thesis that the "ultimate reason for the need for religion is man's infantile helplessness," Freud writes in his book:

> But man's helplessness remains and along with it his longing for his father, and the gods. The gods retain their threefold task: they must exorcize the terrors of nature, they must reconcile men to the cruelty of Fate, particularly as it is shown in death, and they must compensate them for the sufferings and privations which a civilized life in common has imposed on them.
> (Freud, 1927, p. 17)

The importance of the first task diminishes with increasing knowledge and mastery of nature. However, the gods occasionally intervene, as if to demonstrate that they have given up nothing of their original sphere of power. And Freud continues:

> As regards the apportioning of destinies, an unpleasant suspicion persisted that the perplexity and helplessness of the human race could not

> be remedied. It was here that the gods were most apt to fail. If they themselves created Fate, then their counsels must be deemed inscrutable. The notion dawned on the most gifted people of antiquity that Moira [Fate] stood above the gods and that the gods themselves had their own destinies. And the more autonomous nature became and the more the gods withdrew from it, the more earnestly were all expectations directed to the third function of the gods – the more did morality become their true domain. It now became the task of the gods to even out the defects and evils of civilization, to attend to the sufferings which men inflict on one another in their life together and to watch over the fulfilment of the precepts of civilization, which men obey so imperfectly. Those precepts themselves were credited with a divine origin; they were elevated beyond human society and were extended to nature and the universe.
>
> And thus a store of ideas is created, born from man's need to make his helplessness tolerable and built up from the material of memories of the helplessness of his own childhood and the childhood of the human race.
>
> (Freud, 1927, p. 18)

After discussing the psychological significance of religious ideas and their illusory character, Freud turns to the relationship between society and religion. He deals with the argument that one should not question religion as the basis of our culture without serious consequences, just as one should not carry out archaeological excavations under houses at the risk of them collapsing. Freud disagrees and takes the opposite view, that it is

> a greater risk if we maintain our present attitude to religion than if we give it up.
>
> (Freud, 1927, p. 35)

Freud's first argument: if religion had succeeded in making the majority of people happy, consoling them and reconciling them with life, it would never occur to anyone to question it. Second, the progress of science inevitably leads to the decline of religion. This is not a problem for intellectuals, but it is for the uneducated masses:

> If the sole reason why you must not kill your neighbour is because God has forbidden it and will severely punish you for it in this or the next life then, when you learn that there is no God and that you need not fear His punishment, you will certainly kill your neighbour without hesitation, and you can only be prevented from doing so by mundane force. Thus either these dangerous masses must be held down most severely and kept most carefully away from any chance of intellectual awakening, or else the relationship between civilization and religion must undergo a fundamental revision.
>
> (Freud, 1927, p. 39)

Freud has two answers to the question of the future of religion: an ideal one based on rationality, science, and the withdrawal of religion; but for Freud, the time for the "primacy of the intellect" has not yet come. On the other hand, he sees a realistic perspective in the

> retaining the religious doctrinal system as the basis of education and of man's communal life. This is a practical problem, not a question of reality-value. Since, for the sake of preserving our civilization, we cannot postpone influencing the individual until he has become ripe for civilization (and many would never become so in any case), since we are obliged to impose on the growing child some doctrinal system which shall operate in him as an axiom that admits of no criticism, it seems to me that the religious system is by far the most suitable for the purpose. And it is so, of course, precisely on account of its wish-fulfilling and consolatory power, by which you claim to recognize it as an "illusion". In view of the difficulty of discovering anything about reality – indeed, of the doubt whether it is possible for us to do so at all – we must not overlook the fact that human needs, too, are a piece of reality, and, in fact, an important piece and one that concerns us especially closely.
>
> (Freud, 1927, p. 52)

But Freud does not give up hope: He believes that reason will prevail over religion in the long term:

> [. . .] The voice of the intellect is a soft one, but it does not rest till it has gained a hearing.
>
> (Freud, 1927, p. 53)

However, he qualified this somewhat later in a letter to Marie Bonaparte:

> [. . .] one is in danger of overestimating the frequency of an irreligious attitude among intellectuals. I get convinced of that just now on observing the reactions to my "Illusion". That comes from the most varied drinks being offered under the name of "religion", with a minimal percentage of alcohol – really non-alcoholic; but they still get drunk on it. The old drinkers were after all a respectable body, but to get tipsy on pomerit [applejuice] is really ridiculous.
>
> (Jones, 1957, p. 477; Freud and Bonaparte, 2022, p. 336)

2.7 Preface to the Hebrew edition of *Totem and Taboo* (1930)

Freud had already sent the preface to the Hebrew edition together with the preface for the *Introductory Lectures on Psycho-Analysis* to the translator Yehuda Dvir-Dvosis (1896–1971),[3] who was already working on the text.

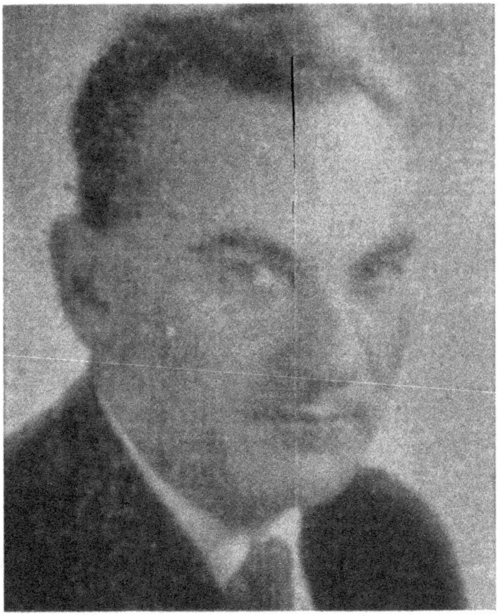

Figure 2.4 Yehuda Dvir-Dvosis, ca. 1935

The editors of Freud's *Gesammelte Schriften* (*Collected Writings*) published the German text in 1934 on the assumption that the translation was "in the process of publication" – according to the introductory note.
The Hebrew book, however, was not published until the end of 1938.[4]

> None of the readers of this book will be able to put themselves so easily in the emotional position of the author, who does not understand the holy language, is completely estranged from his father's religion – as from any other one – cannot participate in nationalistic ideals and yet has never denied belonging to his people, feels his uniqueness as Jewish and does not wish it otherwise. If you asked him: "What is still Jewish about you if you have given up all these similarities with your fellow Jews?" he would answer: Still very much, probably the main thing. But he would not be able to put these essentials into clear words at present. It will certainly be accessible to scientific insight later on.
>
> For such an author, it is therefore a very special experience when his book is translated into Hebrew and placed in the hands of readers for whom this historical idiom is a living "tongue". A book, moreover, that deals with the origins of religion and morality, but knows no Jewish point of view, makes no qualification in favour of Judaism. But the

author hopes to meet with his readers in the conviction that science without presuppositions cannot remain alien to the spirit of the new Judaism.[5]

2.8 The question of a *Weltanschauung* (1933)

In mid-February 1932, Freud had made the plan "to write *New Introductory Lectures on Psycho-Analysis* in the summer as a supplement to the introduction."[6] For him, "the 'New Introductory Lectures' were not an inner need, they were primarily intended to help the Psychoanalytic Press" (Freud and Lampl-de Groot, 2018, p. 74). By early September, Freud had completed the manuscript and the *New Introductory Lectures* were delivered at the end of 1932 (Freud and Eitingon, 2004, pp. 831, 841), the year before the official publication date.

The 35th lecture was entitled "The Question of a *Weltanschauung*" and Freud wrote the following:

> This does not in the least mean that these wishes are to be pushed contemptuously on one side or their value for human life under-estimated. We are ready to trace out the fulfilments of them which they have created for themselves in the products of art and in the systems of religion and philosophy; but we cannot nevertheless overlook the fact that it would be illegitimate and highly inexpedient to allow these demands to be transferred to the sphere of knowledge. For this would be to lay open the paths which lead to psychosis, whether to individual or group psychosis, and would withdraw valuable amounts of energy from endeavours which are directed towards reality in order, so far as possible, to find satisfaction in it for wishes and needs.
>
> From the standpoint of science one cannot avoid exercising one's critical faculty here and proceeding with rejections and dismissals. It is not permissible to declare that science is one field of human mental activity and that religion and philosophy are others, at least its equal in value, and that science has no business to interfere with the other two: that they all have an equal claim to be true and that everyone is at liberty to choose from which he will draw his convictions and in which he will place his belief. A view of this kind is regarded as particularly superior, tolerant, broad-minded and free from illiberal prejudices. Unfortunately it is not tenable and shares all the pernicious features of an entirely unscientific Weltanschauung and is equivalent to one in practice. It is simply a fact that the truth cannot be tolerant, that it admits of no compromises or limitations, that research regards every sphere of human activity as belonging to it and that it must be relentlessly critical if any other power tries to take over any part of it.

Of the three powers which may dispute the basic position of science, religion alone is to be taken seriously as an enemy. Art is almost always harmless and beneficent; it does not seek to be anything but an illusion. Except for a few people who are spoken of as being "possessed" by art, it makes no attempt at invading the realm of reality. Philosophy is not opposed to science, it behaves like a science and works in part by the same methods; it departs from it, however, by clinging to the illusion of being able to present a picture of the universe which is without gaps and is coherent, though one which is bound to collapse with every fresh advance in our knowledge. It goes astray in its method by over-estimating the epistemological value of our logical operations and by accepting other sources of knowledge such as intuition. And it often seems that the poet's derisive comment is not unjustified when he says of the philosopher:

Mit seinen Nachtmützen und Schlafrockfetzen
Stopft er die Lücken des Weltenbaus.[7]

But philosophy has no direct influence on the great mass of mankind; it is of interest to only a small number even of the top layer of intellectuals and is scarcely intelligible to anyone else. On the other hand, religion is an immense power which has the strongest emotions of human beings at its service. It is well known that at an earlier date it comprised everything that played an intellectual part in men's lives, that it took the place of science when there was scarcely yet such a thing as science, and that it constructed a Weltanschauung, consistent and self-contained to an unparalleled degree, which, although it has been profoundly shaken, persists to this day.

(Freud, 1933, p. 159)

2.9 *Moses and Monotheism* (1939)

Freud had already addressed the subject of Moses in 1914. In an anonymously published essay on Michelangelo's statue of Moses in the Roman church of San Pietro in Vincoli in Rome, he had proposed an interpretation of the vision Michelangelo had realized in his work (Freud, 1914a).

From August 1933 Freud again studied the figure of Moses and a year later he began writing the first version of his book *Moses and Monotheism*. In the spring 1937, a first essay appeared under the title "Moses an Egyptian" and six months later a second essay followed: "If Moses was an Egyptian . . ." (Freud, 1937).

After the "Anschluss" of Austria, Freud immigrated to England in June 1938. He was world famous and received an exuberant welcome, including from Jewish and Zionist organizations. He reacted cautiously or even dismissively, well aware of what awaited him.

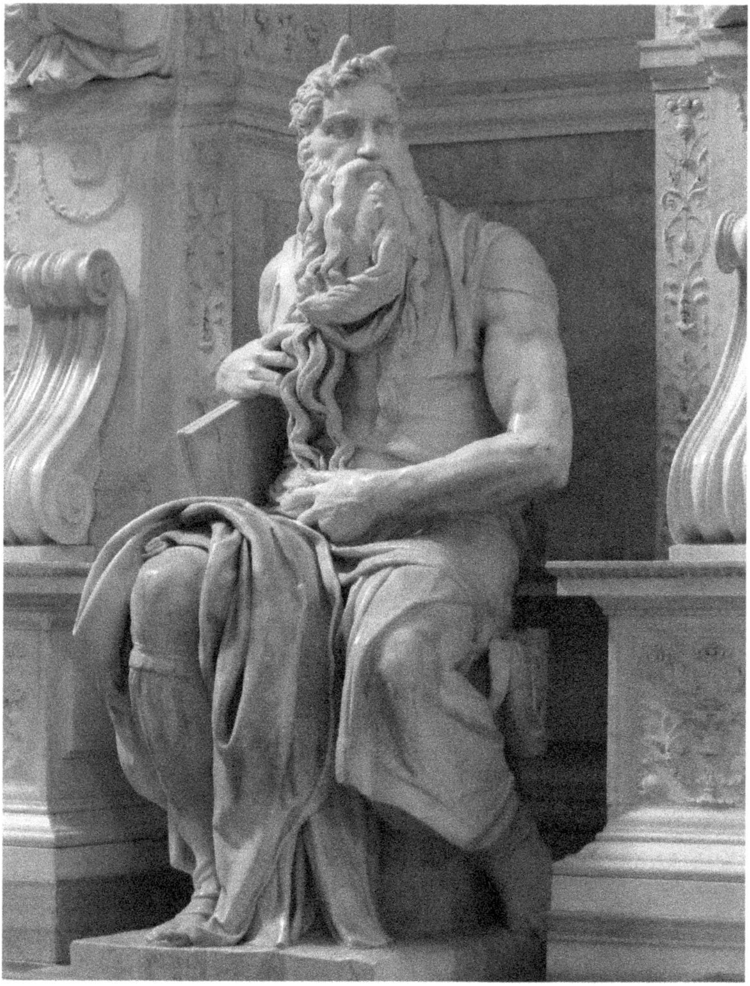

Figure 2.5 The Moses of Michelangelo

On 22 June 1938, two weeks after his arrival in London, Freud wrote to his brother Alexander:

> For two weeks, I've been working like a slave to separate the chaff from the wheat and – forgive the faux pas – answer the latter. Letters from friends, surprisingly many from strangers who just want to express their happiness that we escaped and are safe now, and ask for nothing in return.

> Then, of course, there is the crowd of autograph hunters, fools, madmen, and pious people who send tracts and gospels, wanting to save souls, show the ways of Christ, and explain the future of Israel. And then there are the learned societies of which I am already a member, and the infinite number of Jewish associations of which I am to become an honorary member.[8]

Freud's fear of becoming an honorary member of many Jewish associations did not materialize. A few weeks after his arrival in London, he published *Moses and Monotheism*. It was his last book. His concern that Jews might be offended by the book was justified. Many had warned him before publication, and after the book appeared he received threats and insults. A Jew from Boston called him an imbecile and concluded his letter with the following sentences:

> I read in the local press your statement the Moses was not a Jew.
>
> It is to be regretted that you could not go to your grave without disgracing yourself, you old nitwit.
>
> We have had renegades like you by the thousands, we are glad we are rid of then and we hope soon to be rid of you.
>
> It is to be regretted that the Gangsters in Germany did not put you into a concentration camp, that's where you belong.[9]

But a few months before his death, Freud was no longer intimidated. He wrote about his Moses book:

> It can be called an attack on religion only in so far as any scientific investigation of religious belief presupposes disbelief. Neither in my private life nor in my writings have I ever made a secret of my being an out-and-out unbeliever. Anyone considering the book from this point of view will have to admit that it is only Jewry and not Christianity which has reason to feel offended by its conclusions. For only a few incidental remarks, which say nothing that hasn't been said before, allude to Christianity. At most one can quote the old adage: "Caught together, hanged together!"
>
> Needless to say, I don't like offending my own people, either. But what can I do about it? I have spent my whole life standing up for what I have considered to be the scientific truth, even when it was uncomfortable and unpleasant for my fellow men. I cannot end up with an act of disavowal.
>
> (Freud, 1961, p. 453)

What is the book about? Primarily about understanding the mechanisms of religious genesis. Freud wrote to Arnold Zweig at the end of September 1934 about the circumstances and background of this work:

> For being somewhat at a loss what to do in a period of comparative leisure I have written something myself and this, contrary to my original

> intention, took up so much of my time that everything else was neglected. [. . .] But let me explain what has happened. [. . .] Faced with the new persecutions, one asks oneself again how the Jews have come to be what they are and why they have attracted this undying hatred. I soon discovered the formula: Moses created the Jews. So I gave my work the title: The Man Moses, a historical novel.
>
> (Freud and Zweig, 1970, p. 91)

But only the first part is novelistic. In it, Freud develops the thesis that Moses was not a Jew, but an Egyptian. Others before him had noticed that the name "Moses" was Egyptian, but out of respect for the biblical tradition, no further conclusions were drawn. Freud supports his thesis by analyzing the "myth of the birth of the hero." He believes that Moses was a noble Egyptian who was abandoned by his parents. The legend later made him a Jew.

In the second part, Freud explores the question of "what could induce an aristocratic Egyptian [. . .] to put himself at the head of a crowd of immigrant foreigners at a backward level of civilization and to leave his country with them" (Freud, 1939, p. 18). And Moses not only became the political leader of the Jews living in Egypt, but also founded a new religion for them. Why did he do this? Freud believed that Moses was a devoted follower of the religion of Akhnaton, who originally reigned as Amenophis IV, who ruled Egypt from 1364 to 1347 B.C. and introduced monotheism through a religious reform. After Akhenaten's death, a kind of counter-reformation began, and Moses was faced with the question of whether to become an apostate or to emigrate. A born leader, he did not take the quiet, lonely path of exile, but chose a people he could take with him who would embrace the religion so dear to Akhnaton: the people of Israel. In this respect, Moses also assumed the role of founder of the religion. It was Moses, not God, who chose this people. He wanted to make them equal to the Egyptians and lead them out of bondage, and the new monotheistic religion was to serve this purpose. According to Freud, who drew on the work of Old Testament scholar Ernst Sellin, the Israelites rebelled against Moses after the exodus from Egypt – the story of the "dance around the golden calf" could be a clue – and Moses was ultimately murdered, just as the clan of brothers had murdered the ancestor. The fact that monotheism came from Moses was denied after the murder and attributed to the patriarchs.

In the third part, Freud considers, among other things, the consequences of the murder for the further history of religion. The Israelites' sense of guilt eventually turned into the hope that the deed could somehow be undone – for example, by a Messiah. In Christianity, he also became the redeemer of sins. For Freud, then, Christianity is a late reaction to the guilty conscience of having killed Moses. The generalization of this act leads to a

> welcome means of exculpating God: they deserved no better than to be punished by him since they had not obeyed his commandments. And,

> driven by the need to satisfy this sense of guilt, which was insatiable and came from sources so much deeper, they must make those commandments grow ever stricter, more meticulous and even more trivial. In a fresh rapture of moral asceticism they imposed more and more new instinctual renunciations on themselves and in that way reached – in doctrine and precept, at least – ethical heights which had remained inaccessible to the other peoples of antiquity.
>
> (Freud, 1939, p. 134)

But the Jews did not become Christians because Moses was so strong in their national character that they have always maintained their special position. Freud describes these traits in detail, emphasizing self-confidence, tenacity, and a predilection for intellectual activity. Combined with the fact that the Jews considered themselves to be the "chosen people," this made them an ideal scapegoat and led to the emergence of anti-Semitism. Christianity then blamed the Jews for all social and natural ills for 2,000 years.

Notes

1 Paul Häberlin, Interview with Kurt Eissler (SFP, pp. 15–17).
2 They were Freud's daughters Mathilde and Anna and Ella Haim, the then wife of his son Oliver (cf. Giefer, M., & Toegel, C. (Eds.). (2016). *Sigmund Freud: Die Kalendereinträge von 1916–1918*. Stroemfeld, 122, 132).
3 Cf. the introductory text in SFG 20, p. 17f.
4 Freud Sigmund (1939): מה תאימות בחיי הנפש של הפראים ושל הנברוטיקנים ט וטם וטאבו: ט וטם וטאבו [Totem and Taboo. Some similarities in the mental life of savages and neurotics]. Jerusalem: Kiryat Sefer.
5 SFG 20, p. 23.
6 That is the *Introductory Lectures on Psycho-Analysis*.
7 "*With his nightcaps and robes / He fills the gaps in the world's construction.*" Heinrich Heine, Die Heimkehr, LVIII.
8 Sigmund Freud to Alexander Freud, 22 June 1938 (SFP).
9 N.N. – Sigmund Freud, 26. 5. 1939 [FML].

3 The death of daughter and grandson, cancer, and the end

The first death in Freud's immediate family was that of his brother Julius in April 1858, when he was barely six months old. Sigmund, then two years old, had no conscious memory of it. Jacob Nathansohn, his maternal grandfather, died on 3 October 1865. Freud had visited him in hospital a few days earlier.

The first death of a close relative that preoccupied Freud was that of his father on 23 October 1896, as he wrote to his friend Wilhelm Fliess a week later:

> By one of those dark pathways behind the official consciousness the old man's death has affected me deeply. I valued him highly, understood him

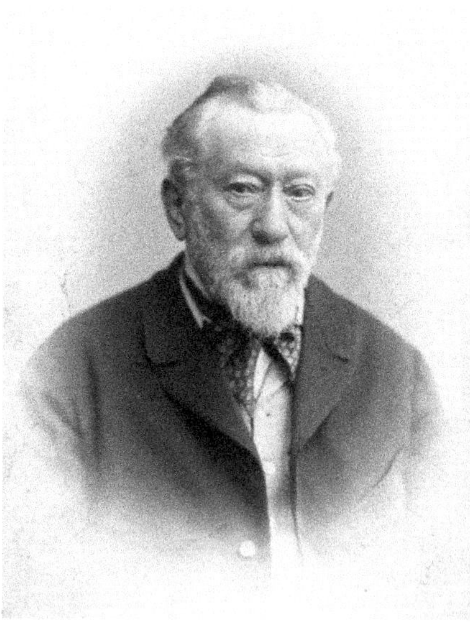

Figure 3.1 Jacob Freud, ca. 1890

DOI: 10.4324/9781003674047-3

very well, and with his peculiar mixture of deep wisdom and fantastic light-heartedness he had a significant effect on my life. By the time he died, his life had long been over, but in [my] inner self the whole past has been reawakened by this event. I now feel quite uprooted.

(Freud, 1985, p. 202)

3.1 "Since I am profoundly unbelieving, I have no one to blame [. . .]"

The death of his daughter Sophie on January 25, 1920, in Hamburg was truly devastating. After Sophie became pregnant again, an abortion was performed and after three days sepsis set in, which led to her death. The day Freud received the news of her death, he said, "One thing is so wonderful that nobody knows yet that

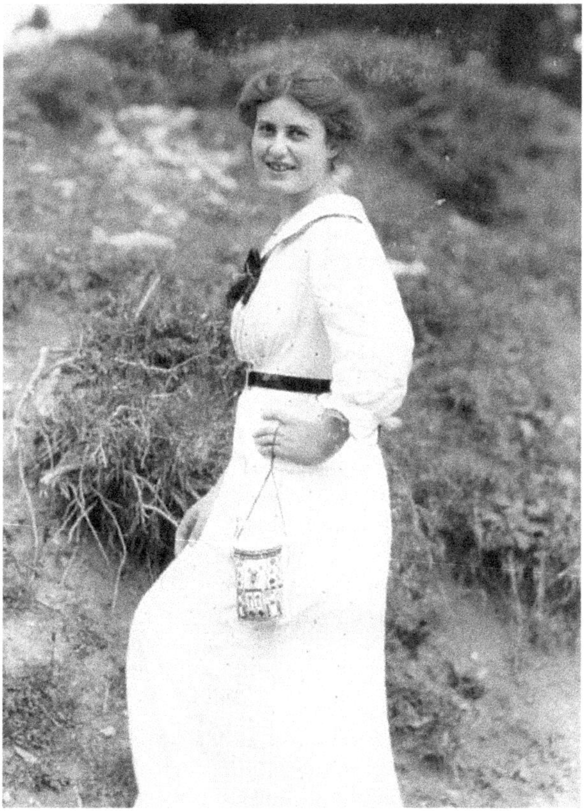

Figure 3.2 Sophie Freud, ca. 1913

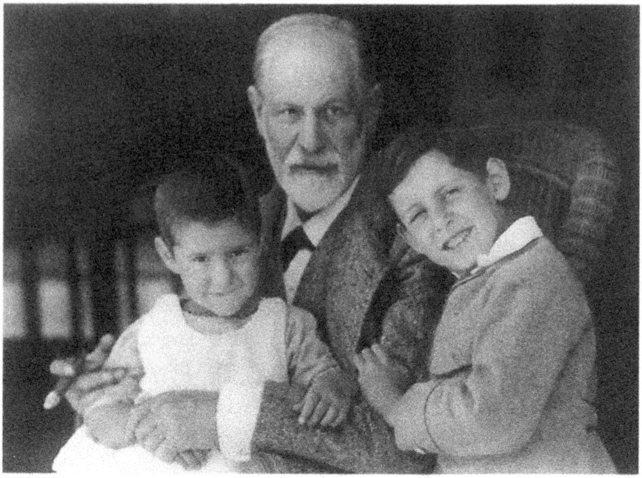

Figure 3.3 Freud with his grandsons Ernst and Heinele (left), ca. 1913

Sophie is dead. Then as people will know, people will come. And I am so glad that I am alone."[1] From the day of her death until the end of his life, Freud wore a small medallion with Sophie's picture on his watch chain. In connection with Sophie's death, Freud expresses his disbelief for the first time:

> The death, as painful as it is, does not overturn any attitude toward life. [. . .] Since I am profoundly unbelieving, I have no one to blame, and I know there is no place where one can lodge a complaint.
>
> (Freud and Ferenczi, 2000, p. 6)

Only three years later, Sophie's youngest son, Freud's grandson, Heinele, died of tuberculosis. The next day, Freud wrote to Sándor Ferenczi: "My dear child died yesterday" (Freud and Ferenczi, 2000, p. 107). And to his son-in-law: "I have spent some of the darkest days of my life here in mourning for the child. I have finally pulled myself together and can now think of him calmly and talk about him without tears" (Freud, 2010, p. 598).

3.2 The cancer

Just a few weeks before Heinele's death, Freud had discovered a small lump in his mouth that he thought was cancer. He kept the observation to himself for a few weeks before asking his then family doctor, Felix Deutsch, to take a look at his palate. Fearing that Freud would commit suicide if diagnosed with cancer, the doctor downplayed the diagnosis to leukoplakia, a thickening

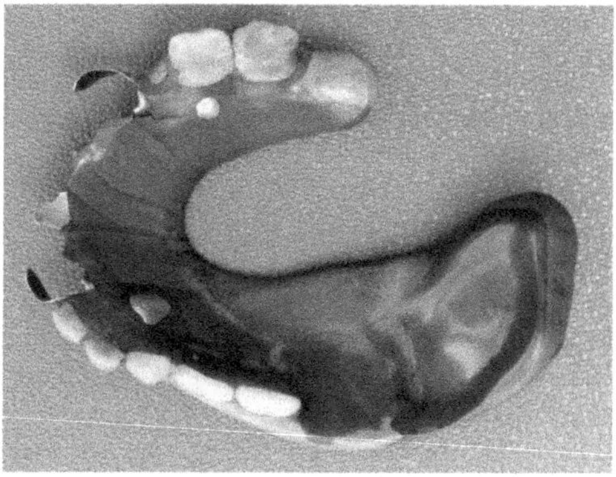

Figure 3.4 Freud's last prosthesis

of the epithelium caused by chronic irritation. Nevertheless, he and the dermatologist Maxim Steiner, who was also consulted, advised to an immediate operation, which was then performed at the end of April by the rhinologist Marcus Hajek – a brother-in-law of Arthur Schnitzler – in such a bungling manner that Freud almost bled to death. Moreover, the cancer was not even properly removed by this operation (Schur, 1973, p. 418).

A second operation was therefore necessary in October 1923. It was much more radical, and from then on Freud had to wear a prosthesis to replace the bones, teeth, and tissue that had been removed (Kazanjian, 1958; Romm, 1983; Davenport, 1992; Freud, 1996). Over the next 16 years, until his death, he underwent some 30 more operations and hundreds of prosthetic adjustments.

But in 1923 it was not clear that Freud would live that long; the doctors had given him a maximum of five years (Freud and Ferenczi, 1996, p. 14), and he was now psychologically preparing for his death. He had two demands of his doctors: first, that they should not give him any painkillers (Jones, 1957, p. 154), and second, that they should help him to "disappear from the world with decency" (Jones, 1957, p. 95).

Both conditions are expressions of his fear of being put on the defensive, losing the initiative, and becoming a helpless object: He did not want to take painkillers so that he could keep a clear head and make conscious and responsible decisions at all times. He even made a verbal agreement with his future family physician Max Schur about these conditions and sealed it with a handshake. Freud now felt reassured and could be sure that he was always in control. If at any point he no longer felt in control of the situation, or if unbearable pain prevented him from working, he could end it himself. For Freud, this contract defined the framework within which he could let his illness take its course. It also left him free to treat patients and to continue his work as a writer, which he did until a few days before his death.

3.3 Freud's death: Lazarus and Euthanasia

In mid-December 1938, Freud received from Rachel Berdach her book *The Emperor, the Wise Men and Death* (published under the pseudonym R. Bardi).

Rachel Berdach (1878–1961) was a journalist and writer. She was born on 8 October 1878 in Budapest. At the beginning of the 20th century she moved to Berlin. There she came into contact with psychoanalysis and became a student of Karl Abraham. She visited the sanatorium in Tegel to see how they worked there. At the end of the 1920s, she began an analysis with Theodor Reik, which she continued in The Hague after he immigrated to Holland. In The Hague, Berdach began work on her book *Der Kaiser, die Weisen und der Tod* (*The Emperor, the Wise Men and Death*).

Fritz Ungar, owner of the Saturn publishing house in Vienna, was willing to publish the manuscript. He sent the manuscript to the *Internationale Zeitschrift für Psychoanalyse* for review before it went to press. According to the rejection letter, the journal could see "no connection to our interests." Rachel Berdach spent the last few weeks before the Anschluss in Vienna in

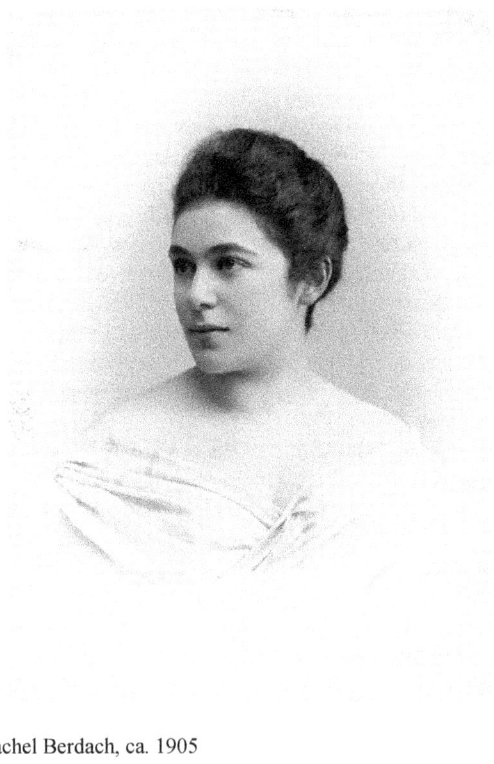

Figure 3.5 Rachel Berdach, ca. 1905

Vienna and immigrated to London on 13 March 1938. In 1947, she moved to Switzerland, settling in Baden near Zurich, where she died in 1961.[2]

Freud was so strongly impressed by Berdach's book that he replied to her after reading it on 27 December 1938:

Dear Madam (or Miss?)

Your mysterious and beautiful book has pleased me to an extent that makes me unsure of my judgment. I wonder whether it is the transfiguration of Jewish suffering or surprise that so much psychoanalytical insight should have existed at the court of the brilliant and despotic Staufer [Friedrich II, Von Hohenstaufen] which makes me say that I haven't read anything so substantial and poetically accomplished for a long time!

And with it such a diffident letter! Can it be that your modesty causes you to underrate your own value? Who are you? Where did you acquire all the knowledge expressed in your book? Judging by the priority you grant to death, one is led to conclude that you are very young.

(Freud, 1961, p. 456)

On 22 January, Freud wrote to her inviting her to Maresfield Gardens on 25 January, at 11:00 in the morning. The conversation lasted about an hour and a half. Berdach told Freud that she had already wanted to visit him in Vienna but had been deterred by the rejection of her book by the editors of the *International Journal of Psychoanalysis*. Freud then repeated several times: "Madam! Why didn't you come? What could I have done for you!"[3]

Freud gave Rachel Berdach a short preface for a planned English translation of her book, which he had formulated during her visit:

> This fascinating book, full of old and new wisdom, glowing with the transfiguration of human and Jewish suffering, the work of a woman who has experienced and understood much of life, should find a circle of readers in our difficult times who know how to thank the poet for her gift.[4]

What is Rachel Berdach's book about?

The story is set in the 13th century. The main characters are Emperor Friedrich II and Rabbi Jacob Charif Ben Aron, between whose death and burial the crucial dialogues of the book take place. For example, an Arab doctor explains to a bishop why he finds the biblical story of the resurrection of Lazarus so terrible and repulsive. It is terrible to have to face death a second time. After his resurrection, Lazarus was condemned to live with the knowledge of what comes after death.

In Rachel Berdach's book, however, there is a second moment that stands out and has a parallel – again related to death: The Hohenstaufen emperor had been excommunicated for making a truce with the Mohammedans after his crusade. Frederick II asked a bishop, who was a close friend of his, if he would give him the last rites. The bishop gave his promise, which he kept. Freud had made a similar promise to his family doctor, Max Schur: if the pain he was suffering as a result of his jaw cancer and more than 30 operations became unbearable, his doctor would give him relief by administering a lethal injection. Freud's doctor made this promise and kept it, as did the bishop to Staufer.[5] Three weeks before his death, in early September 1939, Freud began again with Balzac's book *La peau de chagrin*. It was his last reading. The hero of the novel is a man determined to commit suicide who makes a pact with a magical shagreen leather that promises to grant his wishes in exchange for shortening his life.

Freud's decision to determine the time of his own death was influenced by his attitude towards faith and religion. It was always important for Freud to remain in control. He delegated very little, and even during his travels he received daily reports on what was going on at home and also gave instructions from the road. He did not want to leave the circumstances of his death to "fate" or, like most believers, to a god.

Notes

1 Interview with Hans Lampl by Kurt Eissler, 1953 (SFP).
2 Cf. on Berdach also Toegel, C. (2017). Rachel Berdach und Sigmund Freud: Zum Schicksal eines "Vorworts". *Kleine Texte zur Freud-Biographik, 2017–01*. http://www.freud-biographik.de/2017-01%20-%20Rachel%20Berdach%20und%20Sigmund%20Freud.%20Zum%20Schicksal%20eines%20Vorworts.pdf.
3 Interview by Kurt Eissler with Rachel Berdach, p. 7 (SFP).
4 Correspondence with Rachel Berdach (SFP).
5 Josefine Stross (1901–1995) may also have been involved in the fulfilment of the promise, see Molnar, M. (2023). *Death in the Library* (manuscript) and Nobus, D. (forthcoming). *Freud in the Margins: Rethinking the History of Psychoanalysis*. New York: Columbia University Press.

4 Religion, politics, and society

Freud was interested in politics, current events, and history throughout his life. At the age of eight he read *Consulate and Empire* (Freud, 1900, p. 197) by Adolphe Thiers. At the age of ten, he witnessed the arrival of wounded soldiers from the Prussian-Austrian War at Vienna's Nordbahnhof railway station, prompting his class to tease out charpie, a medical dressing material made from torn linen fibers, which was formerly used as a wound dressing. And in the fall of 1870, he used maps to study the course of the Franco-Prussian War (Freud-Bernays, 2004, pp. 215–217).

As an adult, he voted Social Democratic, regularly read the daily newspapers, and commented on important political events in his letters. In Freud's surviving calendar entries and diary entries, he noted important dates of current events (Freud, 1996, 2016).

Of course, Freud was also interested in religion in politics and public life. In particular, the Roman Catholic Church that played an important role for Freud and psychoanalysis.

4.1 "Father Schmidt. . . a confidant of the Pope"

Freud first formulated his position on the Vatican during his first visit to Rome in September 1901, writing to Wilhelm Fliess:

> It was overwhelming for me too and, as you know, know, the fulfillment of a long-cherished wish. But while I was totally and undisturbedly absorbed in antiquity I found I could not freely enjoy the second [the medieval, Christian] Rome; the atmosphere troubled me. I found it difficult to tolerate the lie concerning man's redemption, which raises its head to high heaven.
>
> (Freud, 1985, p. 449)

The "second Rome" represented the period between the 5th and 15th centuries, when the Patriarch of Constantinople was the head of Orthodox Christianity and the Pope of Catholic Christianity. Freud later even had a dream

DOI: 10.4324/9781003674047-4

about the Pope. While on vacation in San Martino di Castrozza, Tyrol, in the summer of 1913, he had the following dream:

> One morning at the height of summer, while I was staying at a mountain resort in the Tyrol, I woke up knowing I had had a dream that the Pope was dead. I failed to interpret this dream – a non-visual one – and only remembered as part of its basis that I had read in a newspaper a short time before that his Holiness was suffering from a slight indisposition. In the course of the morning, however, my wife asked me if I had heard the frightful noise made by the pealing of bells that morning. I had been quite unaware of them, but I now understood my dream. It had been a reaction on the part of my need for sleep to the noise with which the pious Tyrolese had been trying to wake me. I had taken my revenge on them by drawing the inference which formed the content of the dream, and I had then continued my sleep without paying any more attention to the noise.
>
> (Freud, 1900, p. 232)

At that time, Father Wilhelm Schmidt (1868–1953) had already begun to develop activities in Austria. In 1906, Father Schmidt founded *Anthropos*, an international journal for the study of peoples and languages. And in 1912

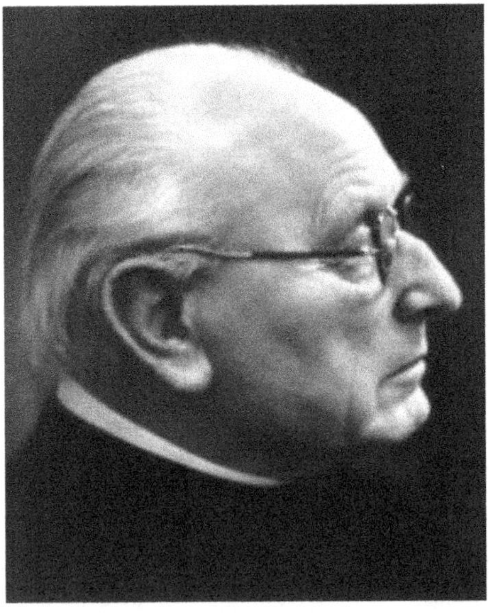

Figure 4.1 Wilhelm Schmidt, ca. 1918

appeared the first volume of his 12-volume work *Der Ursprung der Gottesidee. Eine historisch-kritische und positive Studie* (*The Origin of the Concept of God. A historical-critical and positive study*). During World War I, he served as a field chaplain to Emperor Karl I. In 1921, he became a lecturer in the Department of Anthropology and Ethnography at the University of Vienna. In 1925 Schmidt was called to the Vatican, where he founded the Museo Missionario-Etnologico in 1927. From 1931 he was also director of the Anthropos Institute in Mödling near Vienna.

Schmidt sharply criticized the French historian of religion Salomon Reinach (1858–1932). Freud, on the other hand, held Reinach's work in high esteem, had read his major works thoroughly, commented on them extensively, and cited them repeatedly in his writings. Finally, Father Schmidt was also an anti-Semite, and at Christmas 1933 he called for Jewish businesses to be boycotted (see also Pape, 2009).

Also in 1933, the Vatican began proceedings to ban the second edition of the book *Elementi di Psicoanalisi* by Edoardo Weiss (1888–1967). This book had done much to popularize psychoanalysis in Italy. Freud suspected that "Father Schmidt" was behind the action:

> My good friend Edoardo Weiss has founded a psychoanalytical group in Rome and published several numbers of a Rivista Italiana di Psicoanalisis. Suddenly this publication was prohibited and although Weiss had direct access to Mussolini and had received a promise of help from him, the ban could not be lifted. It is said to have come direct from the Vatican and Pater Schmidt to have been responsible for it. Now, any publication of mine will be sure to attract a certain amount of attention, which will not escape the notice of this inimical priest. Thus we might be risking a ban on psychoanalysis in Vienna and the suspension of all our publications here.
>
> (Freud and Zweig, 1970, p. 9)

But Freud was wrong here. Although the process of banning the book was certainly in the spirit of Father Schmidt, he had nothing to do with it. The proceedings were dropped in 1934 because the Fascist Italian authorities had already banned the *Rivista italiana di psicoanalisi* in late 1933. (Rohrbacher, 2020)

Freud described Father Schmidt's activities as follows:

> They say that the politics of our country are determined by one Pater Schmidt, who lives in St. Gabriel near Mödling. He is a confidant of the Pope, and unfortunately he himself is an ethnologist and a student of comparative religion, whose books make no secret of his abhorrence of analysis and especially of my totem theory.
>
> (Freud and Zweig, 1970, p. 91)

At the beginning of 1935, however, Freud was still under the illusion that "only this Catholicism [. . .] protects us against Nazism." For this reason, he refrained from making public statements critical of the Catholic Church. To Lou Andreas-Salomé in this context:

> The strength of religion lies not in its material, but in its historical truth. And now you see, Lou, this formula, which holds so great a fascination for me, cannot be publicly expressed in Austria today, without bringing down upon us a state prohibition of analysis on the part of the ruling Catholic authority.
>
> (Freud and Andreas-Salomé, 1963, p. 204)

Freud's harshest condemnation of the Vatican dates from 1937, when the French psychoanalyst René Laforgue (1894–1962) visited Freud on 14 November and tried to persuade him to emigrate because of the danger of a possible occupation of Austria by Hitler's Germany. Freud replied:

> "The Nazis? I am not afraid of them. Help me rather to combat my true enemy." Astonished, I asked him just which enemy was in question, and I heard him reply: "Religion, the Roman Catholic Church."
>
> (Laforgue, 1973, p. 343)

4.2 Palestine: "Sacred frenzies"

Freud followed developments in Palestine with interest, albeit with ambivalence. On 10 December 1917, one day after the occupation of Jerusalem by British troops, Freud wrote to Karl Abraham: "The only thing that gives me any pleasure is the capture of Jerusalem and the British experiment with the chosen People" (Freud and Abraham, 2002, p. 364).

By "experiment," Freud means the Balfour Declaration published on 9 November 1917,[1] in which Great Britain agreed to establish a national home for the Jewish people in Palestine. The rights of existing non-Jewish communities would be preserved. The text read:

Dear Lord Rothschild,

I have much pleasure in conveying to you, on behalf of His Majesty's Government, the following declaration of sympathy with Jewish Zionist aspirations which has been submitted to, and approved by, the Cabinet.

His Majesty's Government view with favor the establishment in Palestine of a national home for the Jewish people, and will use their best endeavors to facilitate the achievement of this object, it being clearly understood that nothing shall be done which may prejudice the civil and religious rights of existing non-Jewish communities in Palestine, or the rights and political status enjoyed by Jews in any other country.

I should be grateful if you would bring this declaration to the knowledge of the Zionist Federation.

Yours faithfully,
Arthur Balfour

(Schneer, 2010, p. 436)

Eight years later, in early January 1925, Freud received an invitation to the opening of the Hebrew University in Jerusalem, scheduled for 1 April.[2] He had to decline for health reasons. On 27 March, Freud then sent a greeting to the Board of Trustees of the Hebrew University in Jerusalem on the occasion of its official opening, which was printed in the official volume of the "Inauguration" alongside greetings from Einstein, Harvard University, the Royal Society and others (Freud, 1925c, p. 292).

Among the speakers at the opening ceremony were Arthur Balfour (1848–1930) and Chaim Weizmann (1874–1952).

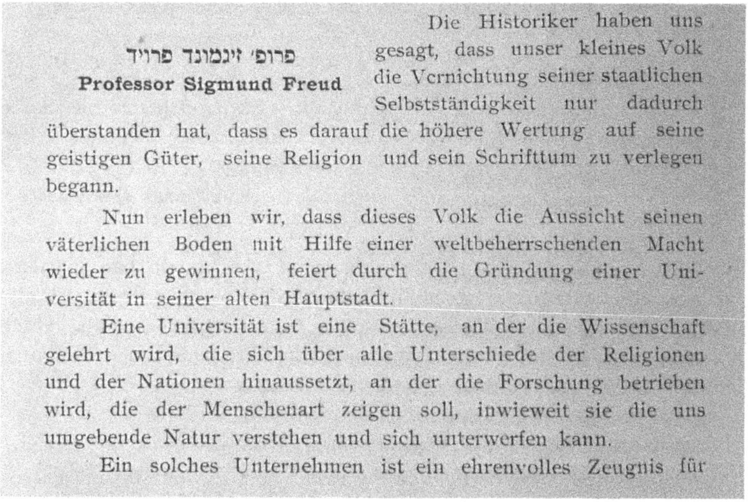

פרופ' זיגמונד פרויד
Professor Sigmund Freud

Die Historiker haben uns gesagt, dass unser kleines Volk die Vernichtung seiner staatlichen Selbstständigkeit nur dadurch überstanden hat, dass es darauf die höhere Wertung auf seine geistigen Güter, seine Religion und sein Schrifttum zu verlegen begann.

Nun erleben wir, dass dieses Volk die Aussicht seinen väterlichen Boden mit Hilfe einer weltbeherrschenden Macht wieder zu gewinnen, feiert durch die Gründung einer Universität in seiner alten Hauptstadt.

Eine Universität ist eine Stätte, an der die Wissenschaft gelehrt wird, die sich über alle Unterschiede der Religionen und der Nationen hinaussetzt, an der die Forschung betrieben wird, die der Menschenart zeigen soll, inwieweit sie die uns umgebende Natur verstehen und sich unterwerfen kann.

Ein solches Unternehmen ist ein ehrenvolles Zeugnis für

Figure 4.2 Freud's greeting address

A few weeks earlier, Freud had written to Oscar Grün (1890–1953), the editor of the weekly newspaper *Jüdische Presszentrale Zürich*, about his position on Judaism:

> [. . .] I can say that I stand as far apart from the Jewish religion as from all other religions: that is to say, they are of great significance to me as a subject of scientific interest, but I have no part in them emotionally. On the other hand I have always had a strong feeling of solidarity with my fellow-people, and have always encouraged it in my children as well. We have all remained in the Jewish denomination.
>
> In the time of my youth our free-thinking religious instructors set no store by their pupils' acquiring a knowledge of the Hebrew language and literature. My education in this field was therefore extremely behindhand, as I have since often regretted.
>
> (Freud, 1925b, p. 291)

On 15 January 1925, the newspaper had begun publishing a series entitled "Jewish Personalities Past and Present." Moses Maimonides was presented first, Arthur Schnitzler second, Sigmund Freud third. Oscar Grün had approached Freud in this context with a request for information about his relationship to Judaism.

And shortly after his 70th birthday, which was celebrated around the world, Freud wrote to Marie Bonaparte:

> The Jewish societies in Vienna and the University in Jerusalem (of which I am a trustee), in short the Jews altogether, have celebrated me like a national hero, although my service to the Jewish cause is confined to the single point that I have never denied my Jewishness.
>
> (Freud, 1961, p. 368)

However, his attitude toward the establishment of a Jewish state in Palestine gradually began to change. In mid-February 1930, Chaim Koffler (1885–1944), a representative of Keren Hayesod, a Zionist organization that raised money for the Palestinian Fund at the time, asked Freud to sign a petition in favor of Jewish immigration to Palestine. The occasion

> was an Arab riot that had taken place in the summer of 1929. The riots, which resulted in the deaths of more than a hundred Palestinians and an equal number of Jews, including those whose families had lived peacefully with Arab neighbours in Hebron for generations [. . .], were triggered by a march to the Western Wall by members of the radical right-wing Zionist group "Betar". They had demanded free access (through the Muslim

> quarter) to the Wall, the destruction of a mosque next to the Wall and the rebuilding of the Jewish Temple.
>
> (Nitzschke, 2015, p. 17)

Freud replied to Koffler on 26 February. He does not believe

> that Palestine can ever become a Jewish state and that the Christian as well as the Islamic world will ever be ready to entrust their holy places to Jewish care. It would have seemed more reasonable to me to found a Jewish homeland on a historically unencumbered soil; I know that such a rational intention would never have won the enthusiasm of the masses and the resources of the rich. I also regret to admit that the unrealistic fanaticism of our comrades is partly to blame for arousing the mistrust of the Arabs. I can have no sympathy whatsoever for the misguided piety that makes a piece of Herod's wall a national relic and thus offends the feelings of the natives.
>
> (Freud, 1973, p. 17)

On 8 May 1932, Freud wrote to Arnold Zweig who was already toying with the idea of emigrating to Palestine:

> [. . .] Palestine has never produced anything but religions, sacred frenzies, presumptuous attempts to overcome the outer world of appearance by means of the inner world of wishful thinking.
>
> (Freud and Zweig, 1970, p. 39)

Shortly after Freud left Austria and arrived in London, he received a letter of welcome from Israel Cohen (1879–1961), the secretary general of the World Zionist Organization, which included a request that Freud help raise money for Jewish settlers in Palestine. The next day, 14 September 1938, Freud refused the request:

Dear Sir,

To my thanks for your welcome to England I add the request that you do not treat me like a "leader in Israel". I wish to be regarded only as a modest scientist and not to stand out in any other way. Although a good Jew who has never denied Judaism, I cannot overlook the fact that my absolutely negative attitude towards any religion, including the Jewish religion, separates me from the majority of our comrades and makes me unsuitable for the role you wish to assign me.

Freud

(Freud, 1954, p. 775)

4.3 Freud and B'nai B'rith

The association B'nai B'rith ("Children of the Covenant") was founded in New York in 1843. In 1889, an "Austrian-Israeli Humanity Association B'nai B'rith" was founded in Vienna and in 1895 the local branch "Vienna" was founded, of which Freud became a member in the fall of 1897. The organization's main ideals were tolerance and humanity. It also wanted to do educational work within Judaism. This explains why Freud gave 20 lectures to B'nai B'rith between 1897 and 1917 – more than to any other association, club, or university.

Nevertheless, Freud always maintained a certain distance from B'nai B'rith. On 29 December 1897, for example, he wrote to his friend Wilhelm Fliess about the second part of a lecture on the interpretation of dreams that he had given to the B'nai B'rith:

> My second and last lecture on the dream is over and was acclaimed enthusiastically by the Jews. Afterward an eager member of the audience asked me whether completely senseless dreams could be interpreted in the same way. This is the value of popular lectures. A physician and colleague could not have asked a more stupid question.
>
> (Freud, 1985, p. 290)

In 1902 Freud attended a lecture by Max Grunwald (1871–1953) on Hermann Sudermann's drama *Johannes*. Grunwald was a rabbi from Hamburg and an acquaintance of Freud's mother-in-law Emmeline Bernays. At the dinner that followed, Freud provoked Grunwald with critical remarks about religion. Grunwald writes about it:

> Following my lecture we all sat down to a friendly meal. Freud acted as the host of this gathering. He expressed various thoughts about the subject of my talk and made several jokes related to religion. He suggested that many Jews resembled Yohanan the Convert: shaggy coats, unkempt hair, mysterious face. Freud preferred the man in the elegant tuxedo to the one dressed like a Prophet. I thought to myself: how far has this man drifted from Jewish life that he can't accept the oriental trappings of his ancestors?
>
> (Grunwald, 1941, p. 119)

In the spring of 1904, Freud gave a lecture at B'nai B'rith on Hammurabi as a lawgiver. He had been inspired by Friedrich Delitzsch's *Babel und Bibel* (*Babel and Bible*) and probably also by David Müller's *Die Gesetze Hammurabis und ihr Verhältnis zur mosaischen Gesetzgebung* (*The Laws of Hammurabi and Their Relationship to Mosaic Legislation*).

However, Freud had forgotten the illustration of Hammurabi's tablets of Law, and Max Grunwald, who was again present, interpreted this error as an

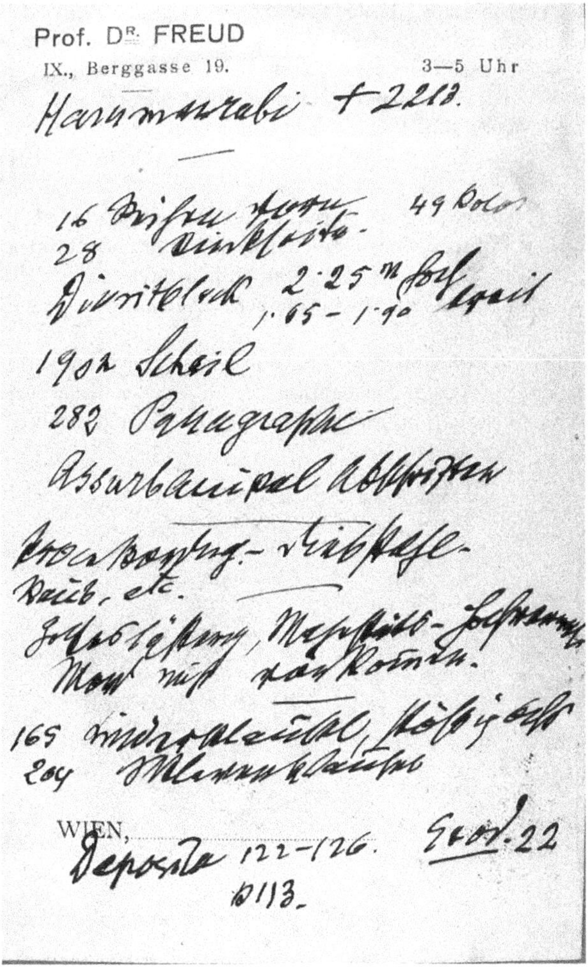
Prof. Dr. FREUD
IX., Berggasse 19. 3—5 Uhr
WIEN,

Figure 4.3 Freud's notes on Hammurabi

expression of Freud's guilty conscience for having held Hammurabi in higher esteem than Moses (Grunwald, 1941, p. 119).

Finally, Grunwald mentions a discussion following a lecture he had given on Jewish education. Freud had claimed that Jews had made no significant contribution to our knowledge. Grunwald then continues:

> The well-known dermatologist, Prof. Salomon Ehrmann, a colleague of Freud at the University, then took advantage of the deadly silence that

followed Freud's attack on Judaism to reply. I was not surprised by Freud's attack since in certain circles in Vienna "Jews without any respect for their ancestors" amused themselves in self-destructive activities. Arman stated that while we Jews perhaps did not invent the generator or the auto, we did give to the world the "Tanach"[3] and with it God.

(Grunwald, 1941, p. 119)

The Grand President of B'nai B'rith, Salomon Ehrmann (1854–1926), had been friends with Freud since their student days. Ehrmann also spoke at the B'nai B'rith's celebration of Freud's 70th birthday on 8 May 1926.

In a speech of thanks read by his brother Alexander Freud said in part:

What tied me to Jewry was – I have to admit it – not the faith, not even the national pride, for I was always an unbeliever, have been brought up without religion, but not without respect for the so-called "ethical"

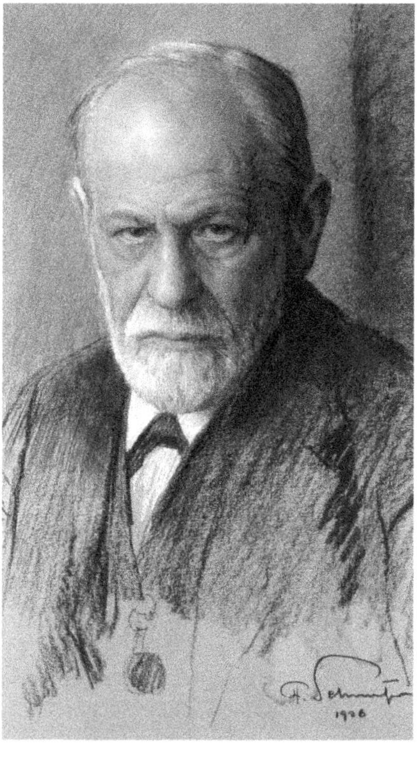

Figure 4.4 Freud 1926, etching by Ferdinand Schmutzer

demands of human civilization. Whenever I have experienced feelings of national exaltation, I have tried to suppress them as disastrous and unfair, frightened by the warning example of those nations among which we Jews live. But there remained enough to make the attraction of Judaism and the Jews irresistible, many dark emotional powers all the stronger the less they could be expressed in words, as well as the clear consciousness of an inner identity, the familiarity of the same psychological structure. And before long there followed the realization that it was only to my Jewish nature that I owed the two qualities that have become indispensable to me throughout my difficult life. Because I was a Jew I found myself free of many prejudices which restrict others in the use of the intellect: as a Jew I was prepared to be in the opposition and to renounce agreement with the "compact majority".

So I became one of you, took part in your humanitarian and national interests, made friends among you and persuaded the few friends who had remained with me to join our Lodge. There was, after all, no question of my trying to convince you of my new doctrines, but at a time when no one in Europe would listen to me and I had no pupils in Vienna, you offered me your sympathetic attention. You were my first audience.

(Freud, 1961, p. 366)

Notes

1 This is a letter that the British Foreign Secretary Arthur Balfour to Lord Walter Rothschild, a leader of the British Jewish community.

2 The invitation probably came about on the initiative of Rabbi Hirsch Chajes (1876–1927). He had been Chief Rabbi of Vienna since 1918 and came from Brody, the birthplace of Freud's mother, Andreas-Salomé, L. (1895). Papers of Lou Andreas-Salomé (LoC). In (p. 87): LoC., p. 184; cf. also Anna Freud to Max Eitingon, 14 January 1925 (SFP).

3 The Hebrew Bible.

Epilogue: Sigmund Freud and *Charlie Hebdo*

In this booklet, I have attempted to trace the emergence and development of Freud's understanding of religion, while refraining from any evaluation. In this epilogue, however, I would like to comment on a statement of Freud in connection with the attack on the French magazine *Charlie Hebdo*.

Charlie Hebdo published cartoons of the Prophet Muhammad in 2012. Shortly thereafter, its editor-in-chief, Stéphane Charbonnier, was "wanted" for crimes against Islam in a magazine with close ties to al-Qaeda. The call was accompanied by phrases such as "One bullet a day protects against infidels" and "Defend the Prophet Muhammad."[1]

But Charbonnier refused to be intimidated. In a radio interview, he said:

> We publish cartoons every week about everyone and everything. But when it comes to the Prophet, it's called provocation. First you can't draw Muhammad, then you can't draw a radical Muslim, and every time it's called provocation for a Muslim. Is freedom of the press a provocation?[2]

In 2015, Charbonnier and 11 other employees of the magazine were shot dead by Islamists.

* * *

Freud always made it clear that his critique of religion was not directed against any particular religion, but against any religion whose "ultimate basis of man's need for religion is infantile helplessness" (Freud and Jung, 1974, p. 282).

Islam appears only indirectly in Freud's work, for example in a 1930 letter to Chaim Koffler of the Jewish Agency. Freud was responding to Koffler's request to support Zionism:

> I cannot do what you wish. [. . .] If you want to influence a crowd, you must have something full-sounding and enthusiastic to say to them, and that does not allow my sober assessment of Zionism. I certainly have the

DOI: 10.4324/9781003674047-5

> best sympathies for its aspirations, am proud of our university in Jerusalem and rejoice in the prosperity of our settlements. But on the other hand, I do not believe that Palestine can ever become a Jewish state and that the Christian and Islamic worlds will ever be prepared to hand over their sanctuaries to Jewish care. It would have seemed more reasonable to me to found a Jewish fatherland on a historically unencumbered soil; I know that such a rational intention would never have won the enthusiasm of the masses and the resources of the rich. I also admit with regret that the unrealistic fanaticism of our comrades is partly to blame for arousing the distrust of the Arabs. I can have no sympathy at all for the misguided piety that turns a piece of Herod's wall a national relic and, because of it, challenges the feelings of the natives.
>
> (Freud, 1973, p. 17)

Freud had a solution to the problems caused by religious fanaticism: In *The Future of an Illusion*, published in 1927, he argued that it is "a greater risk if we maintain our present attitude to religion than if we give it up" (Freud, 1927, p. 35). For the future of culture, that is, civilization, Freud relied on rationality, science, and the retreat of religion. In the long run, he believed, reason would prevail over religion. He formulated this conviction in the sentence: "[. . .] The voice of the intellect is a soft one, but it does not rest till it has gained a hearing" (Freud, 1927, p. 53).

Freud knew that wars have been waged and crimes committed in the name of all the great religions. But he probably would not have thought it possible that the World Trade Center would be destroyed, the management of a satirical magazine murdered, and a French high school teacher beheaded in the name of a religion.

Had Freud lived to see this development, he would have called even more forcefully for the banishment of all religion from public life.

Notes

1 Dashiell Bennett: Look Who's on Al Qaeda's Most-Wanted List, thewire.com, 1 March 2013.

2 "Charlie Hebdo": Parisian satirical newspaper shows new Muhammed cartoons. In: *Spiegel Online*. 19 September 2012.

Chronology of Freud's interest in religion

1858/1859
Freud's nanny is carrying him off to some church. At home, Sigmund preached and tells about "God Almighty."

1866
Freud's father tells his son about being humiliated by a Christian.

1869
Freud reads an essay by Ludwig Börne that sharply criticizes Christianity.

1873
Freud begins to study Darwin and attends Carl Brühl's Sunday lectures.

1874 September 18
Freud formulates an ironic critique of religion, including the remark, "certain holidays are distinguished by a very special religious effect on the abdominal organs."

1874 November
Freud attends a colloquium by Franz Brentano's on "The Existence of God" and reads Ludwig Feuerbach's critical writings on religion.

1883 September 16
Freud attends the funeral of Nathan Weiss and writes about the words of the eulogist: "He spoke with the powerful voice of the fanatic, with the fervour of the savage, merciless Jew. We all froze with indignation and shame before the Christians among us. It was as if we had given them the right to believe that we worshiped the God of vengeance and not of love."

1883 October beginning
Freud ignores the Jewish New Year and refuses to write a letter to his mother-in-law on the occasion, despite his religious teacher's request.

1883 November 29
Freud sends his fiancée Martha a translation of a passage from John Stuart Mill's *Autobiography*, with the opening sentence: "I was brought up [. . .] without any religious belief [. . .]."

DOI: 10.4324/9781003674047-6

1884 May 15
Freud attends the wedding of his friend Josef Paneth with Sophie Schwab. He "was terribly annoyed at the whole barbarism, and that two good people should have to choke down religious hypocrisy at the moment when they were really moved and wanted to be more, and I thought how I could spare myself that."

1886 March 23
In the presence of Martha's Jewish relatives, Freud deliberately violates the kosher dietary rules and demands "cheese after the meat dish."

1886 September 14
Freud marries in Hamburg according to Jewish ceremonies, bowing only to the legal regulations in Austria, which forced him to marry with divine blessing. A civil marriage alone would not have been recognized in Austria.

1886 October 1
It is a Friday and the young couple's first day in their new apartment. Freud does not buy Sabbath candles because he detests religious rituals. Martha is deeply affected.

1889 December 7
Birth of Freud's son Martin. He is not circumcised, nor are his future sons Oliver (born in 1891) and Ernst (born in 1892).

1901 September
On a visit to Rome, Freud is unable to enjoy the Byzantine sites because he cannot "tolerate the lie concerning man's redemption, which raises its head to high heaven."

1907
Freud's article "Obsessive Actions and Religious Practices" appears. In it, he interprets religion as a "universal obsessional neurosis."

1910 January 2
Freud recognizes the "infantile helplessness" of human beings as the "ultimate reason for religion."

1913 August
Freud has a dream about the death of the Pope.

1913 November
Freud's book *Totem and Taboo* is published. Here he develops his ideas about the similarity between the religion and customs of "primitive" peoples and the unconscious fantasies of his neurotic patients.

1916
Freud interprets Sophocles's tragedy *Oedipus Rex* as an "essentially [. . .] immoral play" that "absolves men from moral responsibility, exhibits the gods

as promoters of crime and shows the impotence of the moral impulses of men which struggle against crime."

1919
Freud writes a preface to Theodor Reik's book about problems of the psychology of religion (*Ritual: Psycho-Analytic Studies*).

1920 February 4
Ten days after the death of his daughter Sophie, Freud writes to Sándor Ferenczi about his feelings: "The death, as painful as it is, does not overturn any attitude toward life. [. . .] Since I am profoundly unbelieving, I have no one to blame, and I know there is no place where one can lodge a complaint."

1923 April 7
After a diagnosis that Freud interpreted as a suspicion of cancer, he asks his doctor to help him "disappear from the world with decency" if he is facing a prolonged period of suffering.

1926 May 8
In a speech at a B'nai B'rith celebration on his 70th birthday, Freud says, "What tied me to Jewry was – I have to admit it – not the faith, not even the national pride, for I was always an unbeliever, have been brought up without religion, but not without respect for the so-called 'ethical' demands of human civilization."

1927 October
Freud's book *The Future of an Illusion* is published. He expresses his hope that reason will prevail over religion as follows: "[. . .] The voice of the intellect is a soft one, but it does not rest till it has gained a hearing."

1930
Freud writes a preface to the Hebrew edition of *Totem and Taboo.*

1932 May 8
Freud writes to Arnold Zweig on the occasion of his first visit to Palestine: "[. . .] Palestine has never produced anything but religions, sacred frenzies, presumptuous attempts to overcome the outer world of appearance by means of the inner world of wishful thinking."

1933
In his essay "The Question of a Weltanschauung," Freud argues, among other things: "Of the three powers which may dispute the basic position of science, religion alone is to be taken seriously as an enemy."

1935 January
Freud believes that he cannot publicly express his criticism of religion publicly "without bringing down upon us a state prohibition of analysis on the part of the ruling Catholic authority."

1937 November
Urged by friends to emigrate because of the danger of a possible occupation of Austria by Hitler's Germany, Freud declares that his enemy is not the Nazis but the Catholic Church.

1938 September 14
Freud believes that his "absolutely negative attitude toward any religion, including the Jewish religion, separates me from the majority of our comrades."

1938 December
Freud reads Rachel Berdach's book *The Emperor, the Wise Men and Death*. Among the characters is a doctor who finds the biblical story of the resurrection of Lazarus horrible and repulsive because of the horror facing death a second time.

1939 March
Freud's book *Moses and Monotheism* is published. Among other things, he develops the thesis that the Jews had murdered Moses "just as the clan of brothers had murdered the ancestor." The Israelites' sense of guilt eventually turned into the hope that the deed could somehow be undone – for example by a Messiah. In Christianity, he then also became the redeemer of sins. For Freud, then, Christianity is therefore a late reaction to the guilty conscience of having killed Moses.

1939 September 21
Freud asks his doctor, Max Schur, to put an end to his suffering. After a day and a half in a coma following two morphine injections, Freud dies on September 23.

References

Freud's works are cited according to the *Standard Edition of the Complete Psychological Works of Sigmund Freud.* 24 vols., ed. by James Strachey. London: Hogarth Press 1966–1974; if not available there, according to the *Sigmund Freud Gesamtausgabe* (SFG) in 23 vols, ed. by Christfried Toegel. Giessen: Psychosozial-Verlag 2015–2023.

Aron, W. (1956–57). Notes on Sigmund Freud's Ancestry and Jewish Contacts. *YIVO Annual of Jewish Social Sciences*, *11*, 286–295.

Börne, L. (1868). *Gesammelte Schriften in 12 Bänden.* Wien: Tendler & Comp. (Julius Grosser).

Clark, R. (1980). *The Man and the Cause*. New York: Random House.

Davenport, J. (1992). The Prosthetic Care of Sigmund Freud. *Dental History*, *7*, 205–207.

Freud, S. (1900). *The Interpretation of Dreams*. S.E., 4.

Freud, S. (1906). *Contribution to a Questionnaire on Reading*. S.E., 9.

Freud, S. (1907). *Obsessive Actions and Religious Practices*. S.E., 9.

Freud, S. (1913). *Totem and Taboo*. S.E., 13.

Freud, S. (1914a). *The Moses of Michelangelo*. S.E., 13.

Freud, S. (1914b). *Some Reflections on Schoolboy Psychology*. S.E., 13, pp. 239–244.

Freud, S. (1917). *Introductory Lectures on Psycho-Analysis*. S.E., 16.

Freud, S. (1919). *Preface to Reik's Ritual: Psycho-Analytic Studies*. S.E., 17.

Freud, S. (1920). *A Note on the Prehistory of the Technique of Analysis*. S.E., 18.

Freud, S. (1925a). *An Autobiographical Study*. S.E., 20.

Freud, S. (1925b). *Letter to the Editor of the Jewish Press Centre in Zurich*. S.E., 19.

Freud, S. (1925c). *On the Occasion of the Opening of the Hebrew University*. S.E., 19.

Freud, S. (1925, Feb.). *Brief an den Herausgeber der Jüdischen Presszentrale*. SFG, Bd. 18.

Freud, S. (1927). *The Future of an Illusion*. S.E., 21, pp. 1–56.

Freud, S. (1933). *New Introductory Lectures on Psycho-Analysis*. S.E., 16.

Freud, S. (1937). *Wenn Moses ein Ägypter war . . .* SFG, 20.

Freud, S. (1939). *Moses and Monotheism*. S.E., 23.
Freud, S. (1940). *An Outline of Psycho-Analysis*. SFG, Bd. 23.
Freud, S. (1954). A Letter from Freud. *Jewish Observer and Middle East Review*, *3*(23), 10.
Freud, S. (1961). *Letters of Sigmund Freud 1873–1939*. Ed. by Ernst Freud. London: The Hogarth Press.
Freud, S. (1973). Brief an Chaim Koffler (26.2.1930). In *Nitzschke, Bernd: Versöhnung – diesseits von Gut und Böse. Sigmund Freuds transkulturelles Erbe, Freie Assoziation, 6*(2003), S. 7–21.
Freud, S. (1985). *The Complete Letters of Sigmund Freud to Wilhelm Fliess 1887–1904*. Ed. by Jeffrey Mason. Cambridge, MA: Belknap Press of Harvard University Press.
Freud, S. (1990). *The Letters of Sigmund Freud to Eduard Silberstein 1871–1881*. Ed. by Walter Boehlich. Cambridge, MA: Harvard University Press.
Freud, S. (1996). *Tagebuch 1929–1939. Kürzeste Chronik*. Hg. und eingeleitet von Michael Molnar. Übersetzt von Christfried Toegel. Frankfurt am Main: Stroemfeld.
Freud, S. (2002). *Unser Herz zeigt nach dem Süden: Reisebriefe 1895–1923*. Ed. by Christfried Toegel. Berlin: Aufbau-Verlag.
Freud, S. (2010). *Unterdeß halten wir zusammen. Briefe an die Kinder*. Hg. von Michael Schröter. Berlin: Aufbau-Verlag.
Freud, S. (2016). *Die Kalendereinträge von 1916–1918*. Hg. von Michael Giefer & Christfried Toegel. Frankfurt am Main und Basel: Stroemfeld.
Freud, S., and Abraham, K. (2002). *Complete Correspondence of Sigmund Freud and Karl Abraham (1907–1925)* Ed. by Ernst Falzeder. London: Karnac Books.
Freud, S., and Andreas-Salomé, L. (1963). *Sigmund Freud and Lou Andreas-Salomé Letters*. Ed. by Ernst Pfeiffer. London: Hogarth Press.
Freud, S., and Bernays, M. (2011). *Die Brautbriefe*. Band 1. Sei mein wie ich mir's denke. Juni 1882–Juli 1883. Hg. von Gerhard Fichtner, Ilse Grubrich-Simitis und Albrecht Hirschmüller. Frankfurt am Main: S. Fischer.
Freud, S., and Bernays, M. (2013). *Die Brautbriefe*. Band 2. Unser "Roman in Fortsetzungen." Juli 1883–Dezember 1883. Ed. by Gerhard Fichtner, Ilse Grubrich-Simitis und Albrecht Hirschmüller. Frankfurt am Main: S. Fischer.
Freud, S., and Bernays, M. (2015). *Die Brautbriefe*. Band 3. Warten in Ruhe und Ergebung, warten in Kampf und Erregung. January 1884–September 1884. Ed. by Gerhard Fichtner, Ilse Grubrich-Simitis und Albrecht Hirschmüller. Frankfurt am Main: S. Fischer.
Freud, S., and Binswanger, L. (2003). *The Sigmund Freud-Ludwig Binswanger Correspondence 1908–1938*. Ed. by Gerhard Fichtner. New York: Other Press.
Freud, S., and Bonaparte, M. (2022). *Correspondance intégrale de Marie Bonaparte et Sigmund Freud (1925–1939)*. éd. Rémy Amouroux. Paris: Flammarion.
Freud, S., and Eitingon, M. (2004). *Sigmund Freud – Max Eitingon. Briefwechsel 1906–1939*. Hg. von Michael Schröter. Tübingen: Edition Diskord.
Freud, S., and Ferenczi, S. (1993). *The Correspondence of Sd Sándor Ferenczi*. Vol. 1. Ed. by Ernst Falzeder and Eva Brabant. Cambridge, MA: Harvard University Press.

Freud, S., and Ferenczi, S. (1996). *The Correspondence of Sigmund Freud and Sándor Ferenczi*. Vol. 2. Ed. by Ernst Falzeder and Eva Brabant. Cambridge, MA: Harvard University Press.

Freud, S., and Ferenczi, S. (2000). *The Correspondence of Sigmund Freud and Sándor Ferenczi*. Vol. 3. Ed. by Ernst Falzeder and Eva Brabant. Cambridge, MA: Harvard University Press.

Freud, S., and Jung, C. G. (1974). *The Correspondence between Sigmund Freud and C. G. Jung*. Ed. by William McGuire. Princeton, NJ: Princeton University Press.

Freud, S., and Lampl-de Groot, J. (2018). *Briefe an Jeanne Lampl-de Groot 1921–1939*. Gießen. Hg. und aus dem Niederländischen von Gertie F. Bögels: Psychosozial-Verlag.

Freud, S., and Pfister, O. (1963). *Psychoanalysis and Faith: The Letters of Sigmund Freud and Oskar Pfister*. Ed. by Heinrich Meng and Ernst Freud. New York: Basic Books.

Freud, S., and Zweig, A. (1970). *The Letters of Sigmund Freud and Arnold Zweig*. Ed. by Ernst Freud. New York: Harcourt, Brace and World.

Freud-Bernays, A. (1989). Mein Bruder Sigmund Freud (1940). *Luzifer-Amor*, *2*(3), 139–145.

Freud-Bernays, A. (2004). *Eine Wienerin in New York. Die Erinnerungen der Schwester Sigmund Freuds*. Hg. von Christfried Toegel. Berlin: Aufbau-Verlag.

Gay, P. (1987). *A Godless Jew: Freud, Atheism, and the Making of Psychoanalysis*. New Haven: Yale University Press.

Gicklhorn, J., and Gicklhorn, R. (1960). *Sigmund Freuds akademische Laufbahn im Lichte der Dokumente*. Wien and Innsbruck: Urban & Schwarzenberg.

Grunwald, M. (1941). Encounters with Sigmund Freud. In I. Cohen (Ed.), *Book of Buczacz: In Memory of a Martyred Community* (pp. 119–120). Am Oved.

Heine, S. (2006). Erkennen und Scham. Sigmund Freuds biblisches Menschenbild. *Wiener Jahrbuch für Theologie*, *6*, 233–249.

Jones, E. (1957). *Sigmund Freud: Life and Work*. Vol. 3: The Last Phase, 1919–1939. London: The Hogarth Press.

Kazanjian, V. (1958). Interview with Dr. V. Kasanjian, October 26, 1958 in Boston, Mass. Sigmund Freud Papers. Washington, Library of Congress.

Laforgue, R. (1973). Personal Memories of Freud. In H. Ruitenbeek (Ed.), *Freud as We Knew Him* (pp. 341–349). Wayne State University Press.

Lessing, T. (1930). *Der jüdische Selbsthaß*. Berlin: Zionistischer Bücherbund.

Mill, J. S. (1880). *Gesammelte Werke*. Bd. 12. Hg. von Theodor Gomperz, übersetzt von Sigmund Freud. Leipzig: Fues's Verlag (R. Reisland).

Mill, J. S. (1944). *Autobiography*. New York and London: Columbia University Press.

Miller, H. C. (1924). *The New Psychology and the Preacher*. New York: Thomas Seltzer.

Molnar, M. (2023). *Death in the Library* [Manuscript].

Mühlleitner, E. (1992). *Biographisches Lexikon der Psychoanalyse*. Tübingen: Edition Diskord.

Nitzschke, B. (2015). Versöhnung – diesseits von Gut und Böse. Sigmund Freuds transkulturelles Erbe. [manuscript].

Nobus, Dany (forthcoming). Yom Kippur (1939) Freud, Schur and the Rupture of the Lethal Pact, in: *Freud in the Margins: Rethinking the History of Psychoanalysis*. New York: Columbia University Press.

Nunberg, H., and Federn, E. (Eds.). (1967). *Minutes of the Vienna Psychoanalytic Society, 1908–1910*. International University Press.

Paneth, J. (2007). *Vita Nuova. Ein Gelehrtenleben zwischen Nietsche und Freud*. Ed. by Wilhelm Hemecker. Graz: Leykam Buchverlag.

Pape, C. (2009). Wilhelm Schmidt. In W. Bernz (Ed.), *Handbuch des Antisemitismus. Judenfeindschaft in Geschichte und Gegenwart Personen*. De Gruyter Saur.

Reik, T. (1912). *Flaubert und seine "Versuchung des heiligen Antonius": ein Beitrag zur Künstlerpsychologie*. Minden: J. C. C. Bruns.

Reik, T. (1915/1916). Die Pubertätsriten der Wilden. Über einige Übereinstimmungen im Seelenleben der Wilden und der Neurotiker. *Imago, 4*, 125–144, 189–222.

Reik, T. (1956). *The Search within: The Inner Experiences of a Psychoanalyst*. New York: Farrar, Straus & Cudahy.

Rice, E. (1990). *Freud and Moses: The Long Journey Home*. Albany, NY: State University of New York Press.

Rohrbacher, P. (2020). Pater Wilhelm Schmidt und Sigmund Freud: Gesellschaftliche Kontexte einer religionsethnologischen Kontroverse in der Zwischenkriegszeit. *Cultura and psyché, 1*, 53–68.

Romm, S. (1983). *The Unwelcome Intruder: Freud's Struggle with Cancer*. New York: Praeger.

Schneer, J. (2010). *The Balfour Declaration: The Origins of the Arab-Israeli Conflict*. London: Bloomsbury.

Schnitzler, A. (1981). *Jugend in Wien*. Frankfurt am Main: Fischer Taschenbuch Verlag.

Schur, M. (1973). *Sigmund Freud. Leben und Sterben*. Frankfurt am Main: Suhrkamp.

Toegel, C. (2006). *Freud und Berlin* (Orig.-Ausg. ed.). Berlin: Aufbau-Taschenbuch-Verlag.

Venturelli, A. (1984). Nietzsche in der Berggasse 19. Über die erste Nietzsche-Rezeption in Wien. *Nietzsche-Studien, 13*, 448–480.

Wysling, V. (Ed.). (1988). *Thomas Mann, Heinrich Mann, Briefwechsel 1900–1949*. S. Fischer.

Picture credits

Figure 0.1 Excerpt from Freud's letter to Reik (SFP)
Figure 1.1 Church of the Nativity of the Virgin Mary in Freiberg (Photo: Toegel)
Figure 1.2 Freud and his father, ca. 1865 (FML)
Figure 1.3 Title page of volume 3 of Brehm's "Thierleben" (Scan: Toegel)
Figure 1.4 Börne's works in 12 volumes (Photo: Toegel)
Figure 1.5 Ludwig Börne's grave in Paris (Wiki Commons)
Figure 1.6 Ludwig Börne (Wiki Commons)
Figure 1.7 Schönlaterngasse (contemporary picture postcard)
Figure 1.8 Darwin, ca. 1874 (Wiki Commons)
Figure 1.9 Volume 5 of Darwin's *Collected Works* (Scan: Toegel)
Figure 1.10 Franz Brentano, ca. 1875 (Wiki Commons)
Figure 1.11 Eduard Silberstein, ca. 1875 (Freud 1990)
Figure 1.12 Freud with Martha Bernays, 1882 (LoC)
Figure 1.13 John Stuart Mill, ca. 1870 (Wiki Commons)
Figure 1.14 Nathan Weiss, ca. 1880 (Wiki Commons)
Figure 1.15 Jacob Freud with grandchildren Pauline and Morris, 1883 (FML)
Figure 1.16 Josef Paneth, ca. 1880 (Wiki Commons)
Figure 1.17 The wedding menu (FML)
Figure 1.18 Birth entry of Martin Freud (IKG)
Figure 1.19 Birth entry of Oliver Freud (IKG)
Figure 1.20 Birth entry of Ernst Freud (IKG)
Figure 1.21 The "Philippson Bible" (HathiTrust)
Figure 1.22 The commemorative page (FML)
Figure 2.1 The cover of *Totem and Taboo* (Photo: Toegel)
Figure 2.2 Theodor Reik, ca. 1925 (Wiki Commons)
Figure 2.3 The cover of *The Future of an Illusion* (Photo: Toegel)
Figure 2.4 Yehuda Dvir-Dvosis, ca. 1935 (Encyclopedia of the Founders and Builders of Israel; www.tidhar.tourolib.org/tidhar/view/8/3055)
Figure 2.5 The Moses of Michelangelo (Wiki Commons)
Figure 3.1 Jacob Freud, ca. 1890 (FML)
Figure 3.2 Sophie Freud, ca. 1913 (FML)

Figure 3.3 Freud with his grandsons Ernst and Heinele, ca. 1913 (FML)
Figure 3.4 Freud's last prosthesis (FML)
Figure 3.5 Rachel Berdach, ca. 1905 (http://www.centropa.org/photo/rachel-berdach)
Figure 4.1 Wilhelm Schmidt, ca. 1918 (Wiki Commons)
Figure 4.2 Freud's greeting address (Scan: Toegel)
Figure 4.3 Freud's notes on Hammurabi (SFP)
Figure 4.4 Freud 1926, etching by Ferdinand Schmutzer (FML)

Abbreviations

FML	Freud Museum London
IKG	Israelitische Kultusgemeinde Wien
LoC	Library of Congress
SFG	Sigmund Freud Gesamtausgabe. 23. Bände. Hg. von Christfried Toegel. Giessen: Psychosozial-Verlag 2015–2024
SFP	Sigmund Freud Papers in the Manuscript Division of the Library of Congress

Index